Out of the Shadows

Out of the Shadows

A Cornucopia from the Psychedelic Press

Edited by Robert Dickins and Tim Read

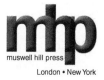

muswell hill press

London • New York

First published by Muswell Hill Press, London, 2015

www.muswellhillpress.co.uk.

British Library CIP Data available
ISBN: 978-1-908995-18-6
Printed in Great Britain

Contents

Foreword

To use the clichés of the times, we psychedelic enthusiasts have gone from Revolution to Renaissance in less than 50 years. In between, I am told, were huge grey patches where many people were unable score any acid; neither scientist, psychonaut, nor hippie alike. If it were not for the magickal workings of a handful of insurrectionary alchemists, the Head's flame would have gone out completely and gone the way of Soma.

Some forty or so years later, as science and the media once again begin to turn their gaze more heavily toward the psychedelic substance group, something remarkable has happened: the manner in which psychedelics can be discussed has multiplied, and their curiosity revealed, beyond question, to have never been the law's naïve black and white approach.

Quite rightly, psychedelics will now never simply be a 'dangerous tool' of social manipulation and neither just humble, psychiatric medicines, they can be *both*, and a million other imaginative things besides. This is, after all, a renaissance – the production of new invention based on the romantic seduction of the past.

Today we stand within the context of an ever-growing psychedelic territory, in which lessons grapple endlessly with history, even as new fields are opened. Over the past three years the *Psychedelic Press UK* journal has documented the great diversity and insight of the psychedelic laboratory, academy, and culture. The often inexplicable heart of which – the psychedelic experience – drives the curiosity of the tripper, the doctor, the shaman, and the psychonaut. All of whom, to use a Bernard Kops line, must 'dance naked in the room'.

This collection is not only a showcase for the renaissance, and the brilliant thinkers and writers who contribute toward it, it is also a critique of the revolution, and provides a range of dazzling gateways into imagining the place of psychedelic substances in modern culture. And, I hope, will help generate the much-desired realisation that psychedelics have an important role to play in today's world.

Robert Dickins

Introduction

We are experiencing a remarkable renaissance of interest into the scientific research of psychedelic substances. Research into their clinical and therapeutic use is gathering real momentum, the media and general public are increasingly informed about these advances and some of the traditional misinformation and stereotypes are being reversed. There is compelling evidence that psychotherapy augmented by psychedelics, such as MDMA for people with post traumatic stress disorder, can alleviate suffering for some people who it would otherwise be very difficult to help. These drugs clearly have medicinal value; it seems inevitable that such treatment will become licensed and available although we do not know how long it will be before we get to that stage.

It is not just a matter of swallowing a drug - we know that the psychotherapy involved requires a special training and skill set and it is clear that the mind-set, the setting and the degree of integration are absolutely essential to the therapeutic outcome. As the psychiatrist Humphrey Osmond said:

> *Psychedelics are the mindcraft of the noosphere. Like spacecraft, mindcraft must be used with crews who are well trained, with ground staff of high ability, planning operations and monitoring progress. It is not just a matter of shooting rockets off into space and hoping for the best.*

There are five psychiatrists contributing to this volume. Among them are Stanislav Grof, the pioneer of LSD psychotherapy until its use was criminalised in the mid 1960s, Rick Strassman, who started the second era of psychedelic research with his DMT studies in the early 1990s and Ben Sessa, a leader of the current research effort.

Some people use these substances with the explicit aim of psychospiritual maturation but mostly they are used recreationally. The use of psychedelics as cultural drivers and creativity enhancers has shaped art, literature, music, our spiritual life and the development of our collective psyche. It seems likely that psychedelic agents have profoundly influenced the evolution of our most important civilisations. The use of *Soma* by the early Indo-Iranian peoples was immortalised in the Sanskrit Vedas, while the use of the psychoactive drink *Kykeon* in the Eleusinian mysteries was an important part of the Greco-Roman world for nearly two millennia.

So we can put psychedelics to *work* for our psycho-spiritual growth but we should not lose sight of the importance of *play,* indeed play seems to be an important part of the work. This collection of papers from the *Psychedelic Press UK* journal seeks to cover the range from medicinal to hedonistic, from creative to the psycho-spiritual. Respecting the traditional role of psychedelics in breaking down barriers and having a meandering course; we have allowed the papers to flow rather than grouping them into sections.

We open to the theme of spiritual awakening with **Cody Johnson's** account of the American sacrament of the 4th July with a firework show over the Connecticut River. In his psychedelic enhanced state, he finds a deeper permanence that underlies our transient existence as he muses over the great questions of the meaning of life and the nature of death.

Mike Jay continues the philosophical theme with the tension between the archetypal heroic journey of the Odyssey compared to the idyll of the lotos-eater – the life of toil opposed to the life of tranquillity and ease. Jay points to the provocative role of psychedelics in highlighting such tensions as we escape the relentless demands of Odysseus, with its parallel to our modern driven lives and visit the kava culture of Vanuatu.

The **Reverend Nemu** takes us to the Amazon, ayahuasca and the richness of the indigenous traditions. Using his rich personal experience, he demonstrates the healing potential of non ordinary states of consciousness and challenges the arrogance of our ethnocentric and cognicentric cultures.

We move to literature with **Roger Keen** who shows how recreational drug use played a prominent part in the work of Burroughs, Kerouac, Kesey and Ginsberg. This beat generation shaped the developing counterculture in combination with other luminaries of the 1960s such as Timothy Leary the Harvard psychologist.

Andy Roberts, an historian of LSD culture in Britain continues the literary refrain with Allen Ginsberg's 'great and perceptive LSD poem' *Wales Visitation* written after an LSD session in the Black Mountains.

David Luke takes up the historical theme with his obituary of Steve Abrams who he got to know at the 100th birthday celebrations of Albert Hofmann – the scientist who first synthesized LSD (and lived to 102). Abrams was a psychedelic activist in the sixties and holds those qualities of the trickster archetype that crucially challenge our personas and the way we choose to lead our lives.

Next up is **Rob Dickins,** whose energy as editorial director of Psychedelic Press has made these papers available to us. Dickins is steeped in the literary tradition and leads us through the role of the ego in the early psychedelic era, focusing on the works of Aldous Huxley and Alan Watts. We are introduced to the concept of ego death as an important component of the psychedelic experience and reminded that psychedelics are essentially playful, naturally anarchic and corrosive to 'top down' authority.

The next section of the book focuses on the role of psychedelics in medicine, psychiatry and psychotherapy. **Stanislav Grof**, arguably the world's greatest living psychiatrist, reviews the history of psychedelics both as psycho-spiritual tools and for clinical research.

Two British psychiatrists, **Ben Sessa** and **Chris Salway** follow; Sessa describes some of the challenges and rewards of the modern day psychedelic researcher and gives a sobering account of media bias in the making of a TV programme about MDMA. Salway looks at MDMA in some detail, taking a journey through the brain and psyche after the ingestion of MDMA, discussing the physiological effects, potential hazards and harm reduction measures.

The idea of ingesting a drug to combat addiction is counter intuitive. But there is considerable evidence that psychedelic induced numinous experience could help reverse the devastation wrought by addiction. Indeed Alcoholics Anonymous co-founder Bill Wilson claimed his experience with LSD played an integral part in his recovery from alcoholism. **Sam Gandy** reviews the evidence in *Trips to Sobriety* with particular reference to ibogaine.

Toby Slater was administered LSD in research conditions and a pleasurable experience turned challenging in the fMRI machine. He describes how a terrifying inner landscape opened up for him. This became projected on to the setting and the researchers; he felt anxious and paranoid and wanted to leave. He settled very quickly after he was given a tranquiliser but his account raises some important questions about the limitations of the research setting and the importance of a therapeutic environment that can support a more complete unfolding of the psychedelic journey.

The next three chapters introduce neologisms in attempts to understand how psychedelics work their extraordinary effects. **Tim Read** in *Archaidelics* suggests that psychedelics do not simply act as *non-specific* amplifiers of psychic contents but as *specific* amplifiers of an archetypal layer of mind, which connects us to a deeper order of being. This leads to a discussion of archetypal principles with reference to Jung, the story of Plato's cave and a tale about the guru who was unaffected by LSD.

Dave King uses the term *Epilogenesis* from the Greek *epiloyi* meaning choice to discuss the enhancement of a person's ability to exercise conscious choice over mind and body. This includes some parts of our function that are normally non-conscious processes and allows the potential to self diagnose and heal physical and psychological ills

Maria Papaspyrou mixes together 'feminine' and 'entheogens' to give us *femtheogens*, which refers to the capacity of the entheogenic experience to revive the broken sacred feminine and filter its essence through to us. Femtheogenic consciousness opens us to feelings of connectedness and oneness in contrast to the prevailing patriarchy with its dominant, thrusting, ecocidal tendencies. We are challenged to change – deeply change – and discover who we really are, away from the social personas that we have constructed.

No one would accuse the former LSD chemist, **Casey Hardison,** of clinging to his social persona, as we see in a remarkable interview by Rob Dickins. Hardison takes us through his arrest while on LSD, his imprisonment and release and treats us to his views on mental freedom and cognitive liberty.

Encounters with apparently sentient entities while under the influence of psychoactive substances are well documented with ayahuasca, salvia, DMT, peyote and mushrooms. The entities associated with each substance tend to have a specific character. If they are not simply hallucinations then what are they? **Jack Hunter**, who had an experience with liberty cap mushrooms of 'an intangible, weirdly organic, world that overlay our own', explores the question.

Peter Sjöstedt-H, a philosopher on magic mushrooms picked in a Cornish field, offers us *Myco-Metaphysics*. This is a trip through philosophy as he seeks to understand his experience with reference to Kant, Nietzsche, Bergson and others.

Henrik Dahl wonders why there are so few visual artists, compared to writers and musicians, who acknowledge the importance of psychedelics in their work. Perhaps it is simply too difficult, requiring high levels of skill, precision and endurance. Visionary artists such as Pablo Amaringo, Alex and Alysson Grey have pioneered techniques for translating their adventures in consciousness into visual form and the prospects for the future look fascinating as new substances become available.

James W. Jesso develops an explicitly spiritual theme looking at the parallels between Sufism and the use of psilocybin mushrooms as a tool for promoting spiritual maturity. How can we use the inner wisdom accessed by the mushrooms? The Sufi concepts of *Rabita* (connection of love) and *Baraka* (grace) may be helpful.

Rick Strassman found that over half of the volunteers in his DMT research experienced sentient and interactive entities inhabiting the DMT world. Subsequently they held an unshakable conviction that what they had just witnessed was as real or more real than everyday reality.

Strassman contrasts this to the *prophetic states* described in the Hebrew bible, finding that the two sets of experiences are very similar. He proposes a *theoneurology* model to further the understanding of the relationship between the brain-mind complex and the spiritual experience.

The last chapter brings it all back home to human relationships. It is a simple story of connection and compassion in post-apartheid South Africa. **About Yellow** shows how psychoactive mushrooms taken for fun finally broke the artificial social constraints between a white woman and a black man. *It is so Beautiful.*

Tim Read.

CHAPTER 1

Fireworks

A Story Painted in Light

by Cody Johnson

Jason and I ride our bikes downtown to see the 4 July fireworks over the Connecticut River. And not just fireworks: this is Riverfest, where families from all over the Hartford area gather to celebrate the nation's independence every summer. By the time we arrive, the 25i-NBOMe is hitting us hard.

We find ourselves at the stairway leading up to Riverfront Park, tugged along by the surging crowd. We lock our bikes below a footbridge, wondering if we will ever see them again, and ascend the stairs to the festival awaiting us.

Just as we reach the top step leading to the plaza, the first firework explodes with a bang, its red tendrils flowering slowly, almost tentatively, across the sky above the river. We join the crowds, jostling for a position near the fence where we can see the show.

I am surrounded by so many people speaking different languages, wearing different clothes and bearing unique personalities and attitudes about the world. We left a thousand different homes this evening, closing behind us a thousand front doors of every shape and color, and took a thousand routes to get here. But we all arrived at the same place to share this experience. Here on the plaza, looking out at the cosmos, we are one. I begin to feel that I am part of a celebration both timeless and universal: the celebration of ourselves.

Words enter my head unbidden, as though scrawled directly across my consciousness by an unseen force: *Festival of Humanity*. That's exactly what this is. We gather tonight, as people have gathered since time immemorial to observe their sacred ceremonies and rituals. This is the American sacrament: we honor our values and our ancestors by blowing stuff up in the sky.

*

The fireworks explode between the river and the watchful stars, leaving rivulets of color that drip like melted crayons into the water below.

The scene is visually spectacular, but what is the point? What does it mean? I immediately reject the conventional symbolism of Independence Day as too parochial, too rooted in one time and place. America's Independence is just one battle in mankind's ongoing civil war for freedom, one mark on the pages of history. I stretch for something more universal.

The meaning suddenly becomes clear. The fireworks embody our struggles and our triumphs, blossoming in living color before us. Each burst represents one member of this human society – sublime, transient, and exquisitely imperfect. Everyone in my vicinity makes an appearance. Parents and children, boyfriends and girlfriends; Latinos and Indians and blacks and whites; people talking, laughing, even fighting. All leave their mark upon the canvas of the darkling sky.

Each explosion charts the course of one lifetime, one human being's dreams and ambitions swelling in a brief breath of life overhead. It is as though God herself dipped a paintbrush into the well of the human spirit and brushed it across the firmament. But She didn't; *we* did. As the brush-strokes stretch and shimmer, I see the full beauty of humanity for the first time.

The mortars hurtling towards space are seeds of potential, little containers of light-to-be. When they explode, the seeds of possibility grow into brilliant blooms of pure light. Once launched, they are bound for glory – just like us, if we choose.

The sky offers a reflection of this festival on the ground. Out there, a collision of souls in radiant hues; down here, the same souls standing in a park, our faces bathed in the light of the celestial ballet. This is our autobiography, mythologized and animated. This is the story of us.

If each explosion charts a human life from conception to death, then this moment – here, tonight, in this park – must exist as a spark somewhere in each fiery trail. The show in the sky not only mirrors us but *includes us.*

For the first time, we see ourselves within the full spectrum of past, present, and future. Every memory that any of us has had, and every event that has yet to occur; everything that has shaped us, and everything that we will ever shape – it's all up there, written in light.

Which is more real, more truly *us*: the gathering on the ground, or the gathering in the sky? Right now, I cannot say.

*

The words 'scheduled' and 'unscheduled' echo in my head. In some ways the fireworks, like our lives, are scheduled – they occur in this moment, tracing a particular trajectory through space–time. If we believe in a deterministic universe, then the fireworks, like all our actions, are inevitable. Their exact paths are, according to physical laws, entirely predictable.

In other ways, the explosions are spontaneous, unpredictable. Where will their paths lead them? How they will appear, and how will they be received? How will they combine with the other fireworks, the other lives, flowering around them? Will they overlap to make even more beautiful colors, or will they vie for our attention, competing even as they fade away? What meaning will they have for those watching?

We do not know until we see them; and it may be some time before we fully understand what we have seen. As when encountering other human beings, we can speculate as to their potential; but only time can tell us what they will truly become, what they will *mean.*

These are the stories of our lives, cast in Crayola colors across the sky. I see what we can *be,* and it hits me. We choose our own colors. We can bloom like the flowers of light that command attention with such power and grace. For the first time, I understand the charge laid upon the living: it's up to us to burst with intensity, to flourish, to make the most of our moment in the sky.

That's all we get – a moment, a flicker of life before we are extinguished. These dazzling streaks of light are all the more poignant for their brevity. Is there anything more precious than a life well lived?

When an explosion is spent, its trails of smoke hang like willow branches in the air, slowly dissipating in the summer breeze. It occurs to me that in the darkness, I can only see the trails of a burnt-out firework by the light of the next one. It takes a new life to illuminate the shape and structure of what came before.

And isn't that how it is with us? We see the legacy of a human being by the traces left on other souls. Perhaps we see a person most clearly at their funeral, when the lives they have touched come together, shining their light on the smoky trails of what was once a blaze of sky-fire. Perhaps there is no better way to understand a person than to hear the stories that are told at their wake – to see the light of new fireworks illuminating their fallen brethren. In each other, we see ourselves.

*

Each firework races skywards, burns bright in its moment of glory, and vanishes as quickly as it appeared. We have barely perceived it before it is gone, replaced by the next explosion.

I cannot help but consider my own mortality, and the fleeting nature of all things. Though we churn and twist within time, scrambling to transcend it, our efforts are in vain. We want to build a legacy, to preserve our species and our lineage, and most of all we want to be *remembered*, to leave some mark on the universe. *Please*, I beg in quiet moments, *let it not all be for nothing.* Or else what meaning does anything have? Why bother living, if our actions and experiences have no lasting resonance?

Nothing is more fragile than a moment, which vanishes as quickly as it comes. And a lifespan is nothing more than a series of moments, dangling like beads on a string, small and delicate between our distracted fingers.

We struggle to hold on to life, to our loves, to everything familiar. We extend our lifespans with medicine and technology, we take photos of our dearest ones to keep by our bedsides, we erect great monuments to our fallen heroes, and we congregate in yards filled with granite stones intended to mark, somehow, the greatness of the people we have lost. We are forever looking back, in history books and cemeteries, in autobiographies and family trees, in ancestral stories across all cultures.

We take intangible things like memories and relationships and, hoping to grant them some stability, try to coerce them into the physical realm. Books, graves, photographs, flag. We build these reliquaries from good solid matter; things we know will last, and fill them up with fragile moments and sacred ideas. We pray that we have granted these ideas and feelings, our most treasured assets, some refuge from the march of time.

But such stability is not possible; no shelter can shield us from the battering winds of change. No matter how elaborate the casket, no matter how thick the granite, the memories of those interred will leak out, evaporating like water from a sponge left in the sun. Books wither to dust and our best flags will turn to tatters in the wind. Our collective memory strives desperately to immortalize, to preserve, to save us and all we know from the erasure of death; but it inevitably falls short. In the end, we are merely looking backwards as we are dragged into the future.

I feel as though I'm floating helplessly down a canyon river. Sometimes the current speeds up and I am overwhelmed, careening through the gorge with no time to think. Other times, it slows down just enough to convince me that maybe *this time* I can get a good grip on the wall and escape from the current, to take respite in glorious stasis for just a bit. But no, the current sweeps me away, silent and implacable as always. Onwards I flow, towards my demise.

Towards oblivion? Or something else? What comes after this life, I cannot say. All I know for certain is that life as I know it will end.

In spite of our best efforts, we die. The bright explosive streamers fade away, and the debris falls slowly to the river, where its final fizzles are too quiet to hear. We will be forgotten; not immediately, perhaps, but certainly with time. All the other fireworks that shone so brightly next to ours must also succumb to fate, and fall lifeless to the river surface: our friends, our lovers, our children. They all die, and with them all memories of *us*, of our identities and what we meant to each other. The spent remains of pyrotechnics float down the river in the darkness, carrying with them the last vestiges of our existence. Buoyed along by the inexorable current of time, these remnants disappear far downstream, perhaps mingling together in one grand mass before dissolving to nothing.

I am struck by a feeling that the Japanese call *mono no aware* – a gentle sadness that comes with acknowledging the impermanence of all things. I savor the moment in the knowledge that I will never see these fireworks, with these people, at this intersection of space–time, ever again. All moments are fleeting, and our efforts to capture and preserve them, including this record, are ultimately futile.

It's not as sad as it sounds, I reassure myself. Life is precious *because* it is fleeting. Death is no monstrous thing to be feared and hated; that is just the meaning we have ascribed to it. My yearning for permanence is just an attachment – a relic of Western culture, which focuses on achievement rather than being, and which is deeply uncomfortable with death.

With only my mind, I have transformed the Independence Day fireworks into a story of humanity. Why not transform death the same way? It, too, is part of the story of humanity. Perhaps it is not tragic that all our moments are transient, resisting our grasp no matter how desperately we try to cling to them. Wind, too, escapes our grasp. Do we mourn the wind?

I am reminded of the mandalas lovingly crafted from colored sand by Tibetan Buddhists, only to be ritually destroyed – symbolizing the transitory nature of material existence. Part of me cannot help but be horrified by this seemingly wasteful, pointless practice. A sand mandala can take weeks to create, and minutes to destroy. All that work, for nothing! How inefficient, how ruthless! How can the monks wipe away their intricate colored designs with such measured calm?

In Buddhism, impermanence is called *anicca*, a mark of existence that characterizes all things in the universe. Because of *anicca,* human life is not just fraught with change; it is the embodiment of change. To live is to adapt, to rebuild oneself anew in every moment. The lifelong process of growth is bookended by the greatest changes of all, birth and death. There is nothing unusual or objectionable about the destruction of the sand mandalas – on the contrary, the monks have merely confronted and ritualized a fundamental aspect of life, its transience.

The more we cling to impermanent things, expecting them to remain static, the more we suffer when they vanish between our fingers. If we can become flexible to change, and accept impermanence as a natural – even definitive – aspect of life, then we avoid unnecessary pain and approach enlightenment. Easier said than done; but the saying must come before the doing.

Anicca has a deeper meaning – one that strikes me unexpectedly, viscerally. Nothing is made or unmade, says the Buddhist doctrine, but only changed. The fallen leaf withers and decays, but not to nothing; its components continue to exist as food for new plants and creatures. It's a spiritual corollary to the much more recently formulated physical law of the conservation of energy: in an isolated system, the total energy remains constant. Though it may change form, energy can never be destroyed. I'm familiar with the idea on an intellectual level, but tonight it really hits me. I finally understand.

When we recognize that a deeper permanence underlies our transient existence, that things change form but do not vanish altogether, then we are free. Though we are merely mortals, we belong to a greater system of life that knows no death. I grace the stage for but a moment, but when I bow out I can take solace in knowing that the show will continue.

I feel like a growing infant beginning to understand that Mama does not pop out of existence whenever she moves out of sight. The realization is bracing, liberating, reassuring. A child can relax when he comprehends *object permanence* because it brings stability to his world; now he can rely on things to continue existing even when they have disappeared from his vision. Reframing my mortality has the same effect. I feel the kind of deep relief that comes only with a broadened perspective.

This is your life, I tell myself; *You are here, and then you are not.* Call death's bluff; spit in the face of mortality. *Live.* Be a radiant sunburst, spilling liquid light across the heavens. Be the one that draws *oohs* and *aahs* from the crowd and gets the youngest ones laughing with delight – the kind of deep belly laughter that can only come from children, ringing out like brazen bells, warding off the ravening darkness that crouches beyond the lamplight. Our strength lies not in the struggle to escape death, but in our courage to meet it head-on.

CHAPTER 2

The Lotos-Eaters

by Mike Jay

The land of the lotos-eaters is known only from a few classical fragments, but it has thrown a long shadow over modernity. The story is familiar mostly from the brief passage in Book IX of Homer's *Odyssey*, in which after nine days of storms Odysseus finds himself beached on an unknown island. He sends scouts to contact the inhabitants, a gentle race who live on the 'flowery lotus fruit'. Some of Odysseus' crew taste the fruit, after which they lose all desire to continue their voyage: 'all they now wanted was to stay where they were with the Lotos-eaters, to browse on the lotus, and to forget all thoughts of return'. Odysseus resists the temptation to taste the lotus; instead, he drags his crew forcibly back to the ship and sets sail as quickly as possible, 'for fear that others of them might eat the lotus and think no more of home'.

Legends of the land of the lotos-eaters persisted in the ancient world. Herodotus, in his Histories, records a tradition locating it near the coast of Africa: perhaps near Libya, perhaps the island of Djerba off present-day Tunisia. He speculates, too, about the botanical identity of the lotos: some believed it be a sweet and heady fruit like the date, and others a wine made from such a fruit. More recently it has been suggested that its flower might have been that of the Egyptian blue water-lily (Nymphaea caerulea), which is now known to have mild psychoactive and sedative properties. But the appeal of the story has always been more mythical than literal. Odysseus was the archetypal man on a mission; the central theme of his story, at the core of his character, is his determination to resist all distractions and temptations, remaining focused on his prime imperative. Just as he was obliged to stop his ears to the song of the sirens, he could not allow himself to taste the fruit of the lotos. Across the subsequent centuries, Odysseus' self-command, and the conviction with which he lashes his unwilling crew to the oars, has exemplified the ideal of leadership and its defining role in the advancement of civilisation.

But Odysseus' steely decision invites many questions. If his commitment to his mission was truly unshakeable, why not at least try the lotos? At the most he might enjoy a few days of contentment before resuming his quest refreshed. Or did he fear that the lotos might be too good to resist? That it might reveal his mission to be less important than he pretended to himself? That if he tried it, he would no longer be able to lead by example, or to convince his crew to make the sacrifices he demanded of them? Did his crew lack the moral fiber of their commander - or was his mission simply less important to them than it was to him? By denying his crew their choice, was he exercising leadership or tyranny?

And what, precisely, is wrong with the happy society of the lotos-eaters? There might be deep wisdom in their serenity; perhaps they have resolved the questions that still spur the rest of us on our endless quests. In 1832, just as the industrial revolution was beginning to blanket the British countryside with factories and submerge ancient rural ways of life under a pall of smoke and steam, Alfred Tennyson wrote an epic poem, The Lotos-eaters, inspired by his visit to Spain during which he saw remote farms and villages untouched by the modern world. In Homer's telling we hear only that those of Odysseus' crew who ate the lotos wept and begged at Odysseus' stern commands, but Tennyson gives words to their lament:

Then someone said, 'We will return no more';
And all at once they sang, 'Our island home
Is far beyond the wave; we will no longer roam.'

Life on Odysseus' ship, in this telling, had become a quest without end, a self-imposed torment that had sapped their strength and destroyed their souls. They had marched, fought and sailed their way across half the world; now, among the lotos-eaters, they had found another way of living:

Let us swear an oath, and keep it with an equal mind
In the hollow lotos-land to live and lie reclined
On the hills like Gods together, careless of mankind.

Tennyson's lotos-eaters are not frenzied Dionysiac revelers, pursuing pleasure greedily and selfishly. They are a collective of 'mild-eyed, melancholy' figures who, like Odysseus' reluctant crew, have seen too much of suffering and death to refuse the chance of peace and happiness. Like Epicurus and the classical philosophers of his school, their ideal is not sensual indulgence or even ecstatic transcendence but *ataraxia*, the state of tranquility that holds no illusions, no hopes or fears of a life beyond this one.

Odysseus may choose to defy death, or live as if he were immortal; but the lotos-eaters know that it will come soon enough - and when it does, the moments of satisfied repose will hold more meaning than the years of pitiless toil.

The myth of the lotos-eaters continued to resonate throughout the nineteenth century, as industrialists and imperialists found themselves, like Odysseus, faced with subject populations who failed to grasp the urgency of their mission or to understand why it was necessary to replace a life of ease with one of perpetual labour. In some cases the myth was projected onto the foreign drug habits of the colonized – the opium-smoking Chinese, the coca-chewing Andean or the hashish-eating Egyptian – and their resistance to modernity explained by the newly-developed pathology of 'addiction'. But there is no suggestion in Homer that the lotos is addictive: those who eat it are not suffering from a psychological illness or medical dependency. Addiction asserts that drugs override choice and free will, but the lotos-eaters have made their choice deliberately. When their fruit is taken from them they do not suffer withdrawal symptoms, only an overwhelming sorrow that their ideal life is receding beyond the waves.

The lotos is a drug, but as so often the drug is the symbol for something more: in this case, the refusal to engage with the world of progress and economic productivity, and to maintain a society in readiness for war. To the imperial gaze, the alternative to engagement appeared only as a delusive retreat into fantasy. In his Colombian ethnography My Cocaine Museum (2004), Michael Taussig quotes a report to the Spanish government written in 1849 by Augustin Codazzi, an Italian cartographer engaged to assess the resources of the Pacific coast. He found a land of rich subsistence agriculture, inhabited by a population mostly of African descent; but their life of ease was, for him, an economic tragedy. 'Plantains, a little maize and a few plantings of cacao and sugarcane do nothing more than satisfy daily consumption, while fish and wild pigs abound', Codazzi complains; after a day in the fields, the inhabitants 'go home to enjoy sweetmeats, smoke, talk and sleep'. He warns that unless these people are forced to work by a police system, the wealth of the colony will suffer. He concludes:

> A race of people, which spends its time in such indolence, is not the race called upon for national progress. Out of ignorance, laziness and misunderstood pride at being free, these people are slaves to their lack of need.

'Slaves to their lack of need' – how strange this sounds to the city-dwellers of the twenty-first century. Our problem is precisely the opposite: once we are subsumed into the global economy, our needs become ever greater and the simple life an ever-receding mirage. In this world drugs are no longer, like the lotos, the talisman and sacrament of an alternative way of living: they become yet another costly commodity, tools that we use to meet the escalating demands of productivity. Most of us are no longer eating the fruit of the lotus but passing each other small packages of pleasure between the strokes of the oar as Odysseus commands us relentlessly onwards towards his promised land of Ithaca. It is hardly surprising that drugs occupy such a provocative role in our society, both fetishized and demonized. Few of us live in the way we would ideally choose, and many of us suffer a world starved of beauty and enchantment. In a society where we must always act rationally and think of the future, the escape from responsibility that these substances offer is dangerous and must somehow be policed; yet they are always standing by to offer us a small advantage or luxury, to give us back a little control over our moods, our energies or our minds.

The European Drugs Monitoring Centre recently announced that they are monitoring 280 novel psychoactive substances that have appeared informally on the streets and the internet in the last few years, and continue to emerge at the rate of more than one per week. Many produce states of consciousness entirely new to humanity, but none will take us to the land of the lotos-eaters. The lotos fruit has no chemical formula, because its intoxicating effects depend on a collective that has constructed its values around them.

When I imagine the lotos-eaters I am most often reminded of the island nation of Vanuatu in the South Pacific, which I visited several years ago. Here, the drugs that have flooded the modern world are largely absent: even alcohol and tobacco are rare, costly imports out of reach of the majority whose connection to the money economy is marginal at best. Instead the islanders cultivate kava, a plant of the pepper family whose root can be prepared to produce a narcotic drink. Kava is at the centre of many social gatherings, especially when different villages or extended families come together. Like the native American peace pipe, once it has been shared any feuds or grievances are set aside.

But drinking kava is also a daily recreation. As the afternoon shadows lengthen, women begin cooking and children play in the surf, and men gather in the center of the village to peel, grate and mash the root for the evening's brew. After the evening meal, people gather in huts to drink the milky liquid from coconut shells. The effect is gentle and euphoric: tongues become numb, smiles spread, compliments are offered to the brew and the host. Those who are not drinking tiptoe around the ceremony with respect, speaking in hushed voices and dimming the paraffin lamps. A kava-drinker may feel the need to be alone, and leave the hut to sit on the beach, listening to the sound of the ocean and perhaps hearing in it the voices of their departed friends and relatives. Many drink every night of their adult lives: kava is not addictive, and they never need to increase their dose. One always sleeps more soundly and wakes refreshed.

Vanuatu, like many of the Melanesian nations around it, had a colonial history as brutal as any on the globe. During the nineteenth century it was devastated by disease, war and forced labour: on some islands almost all men of working age were forced onto boats and taken to work the sugar cane fields of Australia, in countless cases never to return. Presbyterian missionaries banned the drinking of kava, along with singing, dancing and ceremonial dress: they called it 'the devil's root', the same term that the Jesuits used in Mexico for the peyote cactus. Kava-drinking, in their eyes, nourished the natives' savagery and immersion in their spirit-haunted world; only by eradicating it could they realize their civilized vision of an obedient, orderly and hard-working population, their uniformed children processing to church or school at the sound of the morning bell.

When an independence movement finally emerged in Vanuatu in the 1970s, kava was one of the universal symbols around which a fractured people could rally. It holds an iconic role in the culture today, encouraged by the government as an alternative to the alcohol that has brought vio-lence, crime and social division to so many of its more developed island neighbors. Unlike most of the world's traditional drug cultures, kava is not the preserve of a marginalized minority but the pride of the whole nation. It is perhaps no coincidence that Vanuatu remains among the poorest nations on earth, yet briefly captured the world's attention in 2006 when it topped the global table of the 'Happy Planet Index'. As the sun sets, you might almost catch along the darkening shoreline a faint echo of the lotos-eaters' refrain:

Our island home
Is far beyond the wave; we will no longer roam.

CHAPTER 3

Taboo from the Jungle to the Clinic

by Reverend Nemu

Of all the wonderful potions boiled up and blended in the cauldron of Amazonian prehistory, none is more fascinating, to layman and researcher alike, than ayahuasca. With a few notable exceptions such as anthropologist Jeremy Narby, academia does not take seriously the folkloric tale that the plants themselves told the shamans how to prepare them, bringing the powers of a particular vine to bear upon a particular leaf, and thereby unleashing its latent visionary potential. The discovery is put down to trial and error.

In biochemical terms, the *Psychotria viridis* leaf contains the hallucinogen DMT, which is orally inactive, being broken down by the body's monoamine oxidase enzymes (MAO's) before it reaches the brain. The *Banisteriopsis caapi* vine, however, contains compounds which inhibit MAO's, allowing DMT to pass into the brain. Science only caught up with the witchdoctor by discovering MAO-inhibition in 1952. According to sober histories, the discovery was not due to any spirit whispering in the lab, nor anything so deliberate as trial and error. It was a happy fluke, during unrelated research into tuberculosis. Many biomedical discoveries are flukes, including X-rays and radioactive waves, penicillin and Viagra, nitrous oxide and LSD. Mere chance or Promethean serendipity, it was certainly no targeted research program that produced these wonders.

The folklore of the inventors and custodians of ayahuasca also prescribes how it should be prepared and consumed, recommending prayers and songs, periods of isolation and celibacy, and practices pertaining to diet and menstruation. While taboos and proscriptions might interest anthropologists, biomedical researchers and psychologists seem to be less interested - at any rate, they have almost completely avoided researching them. Taboos are followed when research piggy-backs on a traditional ceremony[1], or an individual subject decides to observe them[2]. But any therapeutic effects have not been tested.

Food taboos, for example, are almost universally maintained by *curanderos*, and often their patients; but the only clear guideline from the scientific community on what to avoid concerns the class of anti-depressants called selective serotonin reuptake inhibitors (SSRIs). Consequently, despite the fact that ayahuasca and other psychedelics[3] seem to combat depression, newcomers to ceremonies are invariably interviewed about anti-depressants, and those Zoloft, Prozac and other SSRI's (i.e. roughly 1 in 10 Americans)[4] will not be admitted. This is a theoretical objection, however, which has absolutely no empirical evidence supporting it. One psychiatrist, whose SSRI patients have been safely drinking ayahuasca for years, comments that despite widespread use of SSRIs in the West and Brazil, 'there is no single report of any death or doubtless case of serotonin syndrome that could be attributable to ayahuasca and SSRIs.[5]'

Psychiatrist Ede Frecska, who describes the objection as 'an overprotective but necessary warning'[6], comments that 'the traditional ayahuasca diet... [recommends plantain,] a type of banana, which theoretically would be prohibited by the MAOI-safety diet.' He also notes that the diet 'may serve a very rational function: to increase brain serotonin by tryptophan intake[7].' So why have 15 years passed since the theory was first suggested[8], without a single study taking place? Surely autopsies of rats given both, or surveys of long term drinkers, might generate interesting data?

The scientific community widely publicizes a theoretical objection from its own camp, despite a total lack of supporting evidence; meanwhile it stays silent about traditional recommendations, and neither tests them nor considers them to be important. One excellent study of therapeutic effects, for example, notes that 'specific cautions regarding diet and the possibly harmful combination of medications were frequently taken', but records nothing about the specifics or the effects of the diets[9].

Ever since first contact, when Columbus misnamed New World natives as 'Indians', we have been jumping to conclusions about the indigenous world. We have come a long way, however, and today, as Kenneth Tupper notes, 'cultural globalization opens pathways for the movement of ideas, beliefs and practices multi-directionally[10]'. But if pathways are open, what keeps traditional ideas from breaching the ivory towers of the academy?

Historically, racism has played a part, ever since Amazonian sorcerers (*hechiceros*) using psychoactive snuff first came to the attention of the 'civilized' world in the 16th century[11]. In 1768, Jesuit Franz Xavier Veigl wrote that ayahuasca 'serves for mystification and bewitchment[12]', but the situation improved. Richard Spruce became the first modern scientist to observe ayahuasca use, amongst Tukano Indians in 1851, and the lengths he went to understand the Indians were admirable. During a 15 year Amazonian expedition (begun in poor health and completed deaf in one ear, with intestinal parasites and paralyzed legs), the botanist learned 21 indigenous languages and recorded extensive notes on community life.

Less conscientious was Alfred Simson, who in 1886 described ayahuasca as 'an indulgence, which usually results in a broil between at least the partakers of the beverage', and called his Indian guides 'as villainous-looking a set as ever I beheld[13]'. While Simson noted the failings of his colleagues, he also shared the superiority complex endemic to 19th century anthropology:

Although I will not deny... that many observers are too prone to give merely the interpretation of their own feelings to social and even many natural phenomena, I would wish to be bourne in mind, when savage customs are being treated of, the inconsistency, vagueness, and superstition which pervade the savage's mind and actions[14].

Openly racist articles are no longer published in the respectable journals. But as the diagnostics, cultural assumptions and treatment regimes of pharmacological interventionist medicine supplant indigenous medical systems all over the world, can the academy do more to challenge the ugly superiority complex? Or is it that our cultural artefacts, including our medicines, are simply superior?

During the post-tsunami aid effort, for example, trauma specialists flew in to train locals in PTSD diagnostic protocols. Professors from the University of Sri Lanka wrote an open letter begging that the traditional means by which Sri Lankans respond to trauma be respected - that silent meditation may be at least as appropriate as psychotherapy and antidepressants, for example. Their plea was ignored. The banner of PTSD was newly raised, its missionaries were full of zeal. Pfizer Pharmaceuticals, the manufacturer of Zoloft, organized a conference in Bangkok, and at least one NGO was 'just handing out anti-depressants to people'. Regarding the mission to restore the mental-health system of Sri Lanka, the director of AusAID's comments are revealing: 'Restore is the wrong word, because there was nothing much there before[15].'

If articles published indicate the kind of trains of thought that trundle through the academy, we might conclude that researchers, like the director of AusAID, are simply unaware that traditional knowledge exists. Catholic missionaries gave the shaman his due, at least, reporting that he was conversing with devils; scientists seem to think he is doing nothing at all. And indigenous people, born into a modernizing world, often pick up the prejudice against traditional knowledge. As another aid worker commented, those in the developing world 'are driven by a belief that they lack things, concepts and behaviours that the West can supply... We are confident that we have something exceptional to offer and not the other way round[16].'

Describing the actions of DMT and tetrahydroharmine scientifically can certainly be illuminating, but it isn't the whole story; and the fact that the terms used are generally taken from abnormal psychology can limit the types of questions asked. 'Hallucinogenic drugs', by definition, produce images of things that aren't really there. 'Dissociation', where voices are heard and presences are felt, is a symptom of mental pathology. Shamans, however, do not consider the visions and voices to be hallucinations but rather vectors of information. Many would echo Taita Juan's vocal objection vocally to ayahuasca being called a 'drug[17]'. Daimistas prefer to call their brew a 'sacrament', with all that that entails; but then all terms carry baggage. Psychedelic researchers tend to take set (or mindset) very seriously; but what kind of set do we build calling ayahuasca pejorative names and studying peer-reviewed abstracts before even drinking it?

Ayahuasca is broken down in the lab, but the further one travels from the modern hospital, the more layered the business of administering medicine becomes. A jungle cure may comprise fifteen plants containing hundreds of thousands of interacting compounds, as well as dietary and sexual regimen, counselling, and unquantifiable factors such as prayer and the mighty caboclo Tupinumbá. If this group of factors is too complex to tease apart, and the role played by ayahuasca cannot be established scientifically one way or the other, that reflects a limitation of science, not of shamanism. Of course, every system has its limitations, if we are bound by its terms. But not every system commands billion dollar research budgets and the authority gained from half a millennium of colonial history.

Perhaps lab techniques are incapable of analyzing without breaking mixtures down; 'analysis' is, by definition, separating something into its elements. Even if this was the case though, there are still traditional prescriptions that could be tested, like the Daimista tradition of harvesting vine at a new moon. It would be simple enough to compare concentrations of alkaloids from samples harvested at different moon phases, but no such tests have been performed. Indeed, though a relationship between the phase of the moon and the yield of the earth is taken for granted in traditional agriculture the world over, the academy barely looks at it. Scientists have done their job and criticized the research of laypersons, physicians and others, but rather than designing further tests, agricultural scientists treat the subject as taboo. In *The Myth of Biodynamic Agriculture*, Dr. Linda Chalker-Scott rallies her tribe against the lunatics by banging her spear against her shield:

[The] recommendations cannot be tested and validated by traditional methods. In practical terms, this means any effect attributed to biodynamic preparations is a matter of belief, not fact...

It would be an interesting experiment to compare conventional farms to conventional farms with biodynamic preparations <u>without</u> the organic practices to see if a difference exists...

The onus is on academia to keep pseudoscience out of otherwise legitimate scientific practices[18].

Surely the onus upon academia is to test hypotheses before denouncing them! Untestable hypotheses, by definition, lie outside the territory of science, and scientists need not wage war abroad. If, however, a widely-held theory *can* be empirically tested, but isn't (even though Dr. Chalker-Scott herself outlines a suitable methodology), then why are scientists bringing the considerable might of their tribe to bear on this 'matter of belief, not fact'?

Crying 'pseudoscience', as some scholarly ayahuasca researchers do when the wrong type of spirits draw close, may be disingenuous. Pseudoscience has a precise technical meaning: 'something untestable that is presented as science'. It does not mean 'something that a social group is discouraged from doing by custom.' The technical term for that is 'taboo'. While a taboo may serve a very rational purpose, the grip a taboo maintains over the tribe is so far from rational that it may become automatic. Dr. Chalker-Scott confesses that:

For me and many other agricultural scientists, usage of the term [biodynamic] is a red flag that automatically questions the validity of whatever else is being discussed...

Psychiatrists also maintain a moon taboo - the few researchers that have suggested correlations between moon-phase and psychiatric hospital admissions are roundly criticized, sometimes in rather broad strokes[19], but those who value their reputation steer clear of the popular vulgar theory of lunacy. Moon taboos are also found amongst the Maya, Navajo, Hopi and Hmong. Like scientists, Navajos have theories about why they mustn't look at the moon - if you do, it will follow you and bring you bad luck[20]. But theories like this are just opinions until tested (and everyone's got one).

What counts in science is evidence, and so scientists are duty-bound to militate against pseudoscience. Lunar agriculture, however, is not pseudoscience. Nor is it science, as framed by Francis Bacon, the father of the Scientific Method (though it too may be systematic, methodical and guided by observation). Lunar agriculture, like ayahuasca shamanism, is a knowledge system, and some of the postulates embedded in these systems are testable. But, as Bacon himself wrote:

> *There is a superstition in avoiding superstition, when men think to do best if they go furthest from the superstition formerly received; therefore care would be had that... the good be not taken away with the bad;*

Science should help answer questions, and one of the toughest is: can ayahuasca cure my cancer? Responsible academics tend to reply to the public that 'there is no scientific data about ayahuasca curing cancer.' They might add that there are anecdotal reports. If thinking can effect pathology, as science has established with the sugar-pill placebo, then is this the best thing to tell sick people?

'There is no scientific data' means 'I don't know'; but the *juju* is entirely different. Perhaps scientists might admit ignorance in plainer terms, rather than dressing it as knowledge, or refer the questioner to someone better qualified to answer - an Amazonian with decades of experience curing, perhaps. An anthropologist from Mars might theorize that a tribe that cultivates knowledge as its staple crop would naturally maintain taboos around ignorance. They might also have taboos about knowledge prepared with non-kosher practices (and in science, only Bacon is kosher).

I'm a Daimista with an interest in science, not the other way round (thank the good Lord and all the divine beings of the celestial court) and I observe different taboos. To cancerous questions, I reply that two friends given terminal diagnoses abandoned chemotherapy for ayahuasca, and are still vibrantly alive decades later. A third refused a splenectomy with a 50% survival rate and abandoned hospital medicine for yoga, which eventually led her to ayahuasca. Another Daimista, who did not survive, had announced his impending death two years before his cancer was detected, when his health was still perfect.

These anecdotes, with their teleological pretentions, are neither here nor there as far as scientific data goes, neither science nor pseudoscience. But they make for good *juju*. I've not faced cancer myself, but I did fall very ill in the Brazilian Amazon with a flesh-eating bacterial colony called leishmaniasis, or *ferida brava* (angry ulcer). It began on my chest as an insect bite and expanded to become a pus-filled boil the size of a ping pong ball incubating flesh-eating bacteria. The Brazilian health service phone-line told me in no uncertain terms to take the standard injections, and so did every single doctor and alternative health practitioner I consulted, and plenty of neighbours I didn't consult. Treatment would have been intravenous antimonium tartrate three times a day until it had dried out - at least 150 shots of the heavy metal salt, and possibly twice as many. My sister, a doctor with a specialism in tropical medicine, emailed me links to clinical data and fearsome images: sprawling, putrefying ulcers representing phase one; faces without ears and noses for phase two, when the body's cartilaginous tissues come under attack. She suggested I made up my own mind; so I prayed, drank a dose, and put my question to the Daime.

To put this into context, I was over seven years into a relationship with my favoured 'hallucinogen', which my tradition calls variously 'teacher', 'divine being', 'medicine', 'brother' and so on. Its consistent wisdom over the years had won my interest, and filled my life with magic, with synchronicity and wishes speedily fulfilled. 95% certainty is usually good enough for science (p=0.05), but I could not recall a single instance where my sacrament had given me bad advice in hundreds of sessions.[21]

My visions followed a procession of acquaintances whose leishmaniasis had yielded to injections, but whose lives were still blighted by lingering conditions - permanently painful joints, strange bumps, pathological greed which kept turning friends into enemies. Across the frameworks of meaning that appeal to me, suffering is a common motif, in the Buddhist noble truths and Christian imagery, in the nigredo of alchemy, the shamanic vision of dismemberment and the Daimista's purge. The individual is tempered through trials; and if karmas, sins or imbalances are not worked through in one way, they will manifest in another.

'Dai me' means 'give me', and here I was being given an opportunity to learn first-hand about Daime, which had been my goal in journeying to the Amazon in the first place. My other mission was to finish writing a book inspired by ayahuasca, which touched on many of the issues facing me – disease and health, truth and realpolitik in science, freedom and the philosopher's stone. Bold hypotheses require empirical testing, and again I was being given an opportunity, this time to turn conjecture into lived experience.

The Amazonians around me, panicking that the crazy gringo in their midst would soon be a disfigured or dead gringo, were the terrified human face of something I had researched for my degree and my book - the pharmacological colonization of the body. All over the developing world, brown people are choosing white bottles and white coats over their own medical heritage. While I had given up synthetically-derived drugs, bar the strictly recreational at aged 15, besting the occasional flu with my bare lymph nodes does not amount to much on this glorious battlefield. The lines of my life were converging, the rhyme scheme and metre determined, another line approaching. Why would I abandon so charming a poem half-finished?

Disease invariably carries meaning in all but the most mechanized of cultures; but in academia, meaning can raise taboos. One taboo is animism, the idea that things around us have their own agendas and means, their own personalities (this idea is commonplace in the Amazon); the second taboo concerns 'magical thinking', where life's events have some intrinsic significance beyond sex and survival, and stories have a power of their own. As Justin Panneck put it in a previous PsypressUK anthology, 'substances like ayahuasca, especially in a spiritually-guided container, allow individuals to participate in not only the myths and mysteries that have been discussed for thousands of years, but the facilitation of their own development[22].'

The currency of science is statistical significance. The currency of lives as lived, whether in the jungle or the city, is personal significance, and its measurement is necessarily personal too. A genuinely global trade of ideas is only possible if we find a way to convert between currencies, with projects that span the disciplines. If narrative plays a part in recovery, perhaps the accounts of visions and insights of participants leaving addiction treatment programs might be revealing. Could the presence of a certain narrative theme predict the chances of future relapse? Would different rehab centres lend distinct themes to the narratives – featuring redemption more commonly in urban Christian centres, and battles with evil spirits in the Peruvian upper Amazon? Might certain cosmologies work better for a given nationality or psychological profile?[23]

Doctors invariably answer my claim that I successfully treated leishmaniasis by telling me that a third of cases clear up without medical intervention anyway, and that my 'sacrament' was a 'placebo'. Scientists have come to understand that there is more to recovery than agonists and antigens; the rest falls into the category of 'placebo', whether that is a mother rubbing her daughter's belly or a shaman sucking out spirits. In doing their duty to banish placebo from the lab, researchers also exclude much of the cure. When scientists step out of the lab and into ceremony, however, things get complicated and, as Frecska comments about one project, 'it is not possible to disaggregate the specific role played by repeated ayahuasca administration (the drug itself) from environmental factors.'[22] Perhaps the MAPS methodology could be adapted[24], giving different-sized doses to different cohorts at the same ceremony, and testing for differences in health, lobe activity or antibody production.

'Placebo' might be something of a carpet of rationalism drawn over an abyss of ignorance, but biomedical science has begun to lower lines of enquiry into the abyss, with tentative projects in the emerging field of mindfulness studies. One longitudinal EEG study has measured both increased antibody production and a change in baseline brain function over a meditation program of eight weeks. Meditators, even when not sitting, come to exhibit less activity in the right prefrontal cortex (PFC) and more in the left PFC[25].

From my limited understanding of the PFC, going from left to right would seem to indicate moving away from suspicion and second-guessing the strategies of others, and towards more charitable thoughts inhibiting fear responses. Would it, therefore, potentiate the medicine if the drinker focused on specific themes? Might what Steve Beyer describes as periods of 'sitting quietly in the jungle, with no place to go, listening for [*the plant's*] song[26]' have measurable effects on the brain's baseline function, or even its anatomy? Is there a psychopharmacological reason for the Daimista's repetitive dance and maraca beat, the hours of back-to-back call-and-response songs? Is this why the hymns mention 'paying attention' so frequently, unlike anything in umbanda calls, Sufi songs or Anglican hymns, for example?

My cure, with its diets and daily doses, its poultices, purgatives and mudpacks, was embedded in a context of meaning. The angry ulcer inflamed and shrank as the lines of my story turned around it; and when worms spilled out from it they carried a message about the transient miracle of fleshy incarnation. I fought a running battle with a poisonous snake living beneath my shack which ended when I slammed it in the door, and I defeated another monster in my ceremonies and technicolour dreams. Having ignored the doctors, I consulted a 400 year-old *preta velha*, a black slave incorporated into the body of a medium at a Barquinha ceremony. As drums pounded around us she massaged points on my arm, swished a scarf and blew tobacco smoke around me, gave me dietary advice and prayers, made an offering of white roses. I broke my silence only at the end of the session, and she responded appropriately before I had a chance to voice my question: '*my... name... is... Maria... da... mata.*'

After seven months, having lost ten kilos and one wife, a nurse came into my life, who would tell me her dreams in the morning so we could watch the events unfold during the day. One night she dreamed of smashed glass and of having her hair platted. As we were out the following day, waiting for someone else to finish using the well, she suddenly began clawing at the ground like a maniac. We unearthed enough smashed glass to fill six sacks. Shortly afterwards we visited a neighbour, whose niece came over unprompted to plat her hair. Years later I learned about a sorcerer who had buried smashed glass at various sites there, which had lain forgotten for over 30 years.

Patterns and predictions are part and parcel of both science and mysticism, and this was all robust enough for me. When our twins were born a year after I had recovered, they both had birthmarks where my ulcer had been. My curandero barely raised an eyebrow; a tag passing through the generations is far from uncommon in the context of Amazonian folk healing. My disease, my recovery, and my narrative all came together as a complete package of medicine and meaning, packing an almighty placebo punch.

If belief assists cure, as scientists have proved to themselves with the sugar-pill placebo, then might absolute certainty guarantee it? We know so little about placebo, and any serious investigation of its parameters, as manipulated by masters of the art, would require scientists to stray from familiar cloisters of the academy. But those overly comfortable with familiar theories should take note of the caution Newton issued when he formalized the study of empirical science: 'hypotheses, whether metaphysical or physical, whether of occult qualities or mechanical, have no place in experimental philosophy[27].'

The indigenous cosmos, like the world we live in, is rather broader than any one scientific discipline, which may pose a problem for researchers. Fortunately, however, ayahuasca is not only an object of inquiry but a *means* of inquiry, and one that has been shown to greatly help precipitate breakthroughs in research, in molecular biology[28], and in other fields. The related shamanic claim, that ayahuasca allows the drinker direct insight into the workings of the plants, is the subject of some ground-breaking research. In the emerging field of biosemiotics, the postulates of Peircean semiotics become the measure of communication between species. As Christina Callicott puts it:

> the process of shamanic apprenticeship and the acquisition of icaros is a form of inter-species communication in which the apprentice intercepts and interprets the phytochemical signals inherent in plant communicative processes[29]

The related but distinct field of ecosemiotics can also be revealing. As Alf Hornborg writes:

> ecosemiotics thus does not merely provide a vantage-point for understanding [Amazonian indigenous] cosmologies in theoretical terms, but actually also for validating them[30]

Researcher-ayahuasqueros, with a foot in each camp, need to understand the taboos of both. If we skip the preparations for ayahuasca, and let our minds wander during ceremony, if, as one biomedical researcher confided to me, we usually spend our sessions thinking about girls, we might miss something. Equally, researchers need to be mindful of the taboos nurtured by the scientific community as it emerged from the Renaissance. Some taboos reject arcane knowledge such as animism; other taboos are updated versions of older mores. As Frecska notes, on one of the difficulties of ayahuasca research, 'interfering with the integrity of the human body has been a taboo in numerous cultures and the Western cultural tradition was not, and is not exempt[31]'.

All over the developing world, traditional knowledge is being lost as Western models expand. My Brazilian wife, for example, was brought into this world by the local wise woman, but our own daughters were surgically removed nine months and a day into the pregnancy, just after the doctor's lunch. At 44% of births, Brazil has the highest rate of C-sections in the world[32]. When the new mother's temperature rose a few days later, and everyone was freaking out about infections and antibiotics, I called for the old wise woman. She told me what younger, less wise women had forgotten: a light fever is common when mothers begin to nurse. The status of the wise woman, and of the shaman, has plummeted since pharmacies and tarmac roads first arrived in their settlements. Despite the popularity of 'the shamanic experience', Amazonian shamanism is objectively (as the Marxists might put it) in decline, losing ground to the pharmaceutical, interventionist model in its own territory.

Amidst the onslaught of tourism, land grabs, climate change and all the challenges of globalization, science can be an ally in the battle to preserve traditional knowledge. Physician Gabor Maté, for example, attained excellent results in his Canadian rehab centre by inviting an indigenous shaman to conduct ceremonies; he also raised the status of traditional wisdom thereby. Shamanic techniques can also become the object of study, not just the 'setting' of the study. Musicologist Susana Bustos' research into icaros is a bold step in the right direction, documenting transpersonal effects on the patients targeted by the shaman singing these spirit songs[33].

Adventurous researchers who go native should be cautious on their return not to offend their own gods and break their own tribal taboos. Their gods might require a modest sacrifice, a little enthusiasm, a little animism, a little meaning edited from a traveller's tale perhaps, but we will surely find that the spirits can be very accommodating. The method of inquiry we know as shamanism survived the missionary age partly because the jungle pantheon was able to absorb Jesus Cristo and the virgin, adapted for the tool box of the jungle empiricist. Shamans and priests started to learn each other's languages, and began a mind-blowing conversation that is still ongoing. Jesus Christo, for his part, seems rather more comfortable in his indigenous maloca than in European cathedrals, eternally pinned to the wall. Perhaps a new wave of psychedelic scientists can follow suit and pull out the nails, to free themselves of their constraints.

The time is ripe for more mind-blowing conversations, and for research that is tight on methodology and loose on ontology. Indigenous knowledge, if it is to survive, must be represented, and re-presented, in a language the global north understands. If we pay attention to each other, to our own taboos and those of the other, and to the other worlds that ayahuasca opens up, the loss of traditional knowledge might be arrested before the colonization of the indigenous world and mind is complete, and there is one less cosmology to blur the hard lines of the rationalist universe.

CHAPTER 4

Beats on Acid

by Roger Keen

The so-called Beat Generation of writers and adventurers are firmly acknowledged as the direct evolutionary antecedents of the psychedelic movement, initiating the lifestyle and consciousness-changing experiments that would eventually permeate widely and give rise to the 'alternative society' and all that encompasses. But it's intriguing to note that these elder statesmen of transformation differed greatly in their interactions with psychedelics themselves, and also in their reactions to being perhaps overshadowed by a newer generation when the psychedelic era got into full swing.

The early novels of Jack Kerouac and William Burroughs paint a marvellously detailed picture of pre-acid recreational drug use. In the famous passage near the beginning of *On the Road*, Kerouac lines up his cast of 'mad ones', who include 'Dean Moriarty' (Neal Cassady), 'Carlo Marx' (Allen Ginsberg), Old Bull Lee (Burroughs), 'Jane Lee' (Joan Vollmer, Burroughs' common law wife) and 'Elmer Hassel' (Herbert Huncke): '... Lee in Texas growing weed, Hassel on Riker's Island, Jane wondering on Times Square in a Benzedrine hallucination, with her baby girl in her arms and ending up in Bellevue.'

As well as the ubiquitous marijuana – 'tea' or 'weed' – Benzedrine figures highly as a drug of choice in the late 40s and 50s bohemian scene, and was then available legally in the form of inhalers. Joan Vollmer was an addict and was subject to numerous psychotic episodes, and Kerouac and Cassady used it to fuel their manic cross-country escapades, as described in *On the Road*. Kerouac wrote the legendary first draft of the book in three weeks on a continuous roll of paper whilst high on the drug, and in many ways that act and its relentless speed-driven energy came to define the

spirit of the 50s scene much as Timothy Leary's acid-inspired pronouncements defined the 60s.

Burroughs describes his first Benzedrine high in *Junkie*: 'I was full of
expansive, benevolent feelings, and suddenly wanted to call on people I
hadn't seen in months or even years…' Huncke appears as 'Herman' in
Junkie and is characterised as the archetypal low life bum, a petty criminal
and dope fiend who'd get high on anything going – junk, weed, Benzedrine
or 'goof balls' (barbiturates). It was said that he first coined the term 'Beat',
and he was very much the prototype of the 'wasted hippy' of fifteen or
twenty years later.

Burroughs encountered Huncke whilst forming the underworld connections through which he obtained morphine and heroin, and though the
other Beats used junk occasionally it was Burroughs who became a confirmed addict. Junk went with his personality and gave him important subject matter as a writer, though his general quest for drug experimentation
led him to psychedelics early. Facing legal proceedings after several drug
busts, Burroughs fled to Mexico City and resumed the junky life down
there. At the dawn of the 50s, times were already changing, and he took up
with a new set of young US hipsters. In *Junkie* he describes their new
vocabulary: "pot' for weed, 'twisted' for busted, 'cool,' an all-purpose
word indicating anything you like or any situation that is not hot with
the law.'

In this company, Burroughs tried peyote, and experienced the classic
discomfiture and vomiting on ingestion. He compares the high to Benzedrine but with surreal undertones: 'Everything I saw looked like a peyote
plant.' And when he tried to sleep the following dawn, he had psychedelic
nightmares every time he dozed off. But it was another plant entheogen,
yagé, that really arrested Burroughs' interest, having learned of its shamanic usage and that it was supposed to increase telepathic sensitivity. He
undertook several expeditions to South America and eventually discovered
the Putumayo region where the authentic brujos lived. After several yagé
experiences, Burroughs made the breakthrough he'd anticipated, finding a
new state of being and a feeling of serene wisdom.

These adventures fed into *The Yage Letters*, which Burroughs wrote in
tandem with Ginsberg and which was eventually published by City Lights
in 1963, when the genre of psychedelic literature had become well established. Yagé influenced Burroughs' writing tremendously, in particular his
most famous novel *Naked Lunch* (see 'The Soundless Hum', *PsypressUK
2013 Vol.2*), and the success and wide exposure that the novel gained him
as the 50s gave way to the 60s, alongside his general reputation as a drug-
use expert and connoisseur, contributed towards him becoming a major
counterculture figure once the psychedelic era got properly underway.

Twelve years younger than Burroughs and four years younger than Kerouac, Allen Ginsberg was very much the 'kid' of the original 40s Beat scene, but as he grew in stature and status he soon caught up with his fellows. In the mid-50s he became a leading figure in the San Francisco poetry renaissance, with his poem 'Howl' gaining fame as a seminal Beat work – Kerouac described the uproarious Gallery Six reading in *The Dharma Bums*. And as the 60s progressed Ginsberg, unlike Burroughs and Kerouac, changed his appearance accordingly, adopting long hair and a bushy beard to become the hippy guru figure that loomed large in the developing countercultural scene.

Ginsberg was naturally predisposed towards cosmic visions – through reading William Blake, and through having nitrous oxide at the dentist – so when he got the chance to try LSD in a mental research experiment, he was full of enthusiasm. His first trip was very positive, re-igniting the visionary perspective in a swirl of Kubla Khan and Hindu God-like visuals, and he went on to repeat the experience. In a letter he said, 'This drug seems to automatically produce a mystical experience. Science is getting very hip.'

Shortly afterwards Ginsberg undertook a six-month trip to South America, primarily to take yagé, following in Burroughs' footsteps and gathering the material for his half of *The Yage Letters*. His experiences were very profound, destabilizing and sometimes horrifying – yagé took him far beyond the range of LSD. He confronted death, body-soul duality and the nature of God, but he developed a fear of madness and of entering a permanently changed universe from which he couldn't escape. Ginsberg was very tenacious in his belief in the larger transformational possibilities of psychedelics, and he had the chutzpah to take the bad trips along with the good and continue his quest.

The next step forward came when Ginsberg met Leary and participated in one of his Harvard psilocybin experiments. After an unpromising start with some of Ginsberg's yagé fears returning, he reached a turning point where, after seeing a flash of light, another euphoric vision began to construct. Ginsberg was overcome with a sense that the cosmos was waiting for a Messiah, and naturally enough he felt that he himself was ideally suited for the job. He came downstairs naked and declared himself 'the Messiah' to Leary and the others; then he and Leary began to mastermind the next stage of the psychedelic revolution.

Ever the pragmatist, Ginsberg realised that despite the magnitude of the personal bliss and enlightenment that psilocybin engendered, it could easily be misunderstood by society at large if its promulgation wasn't handled sensitively – exactly the problem that would soon beset LSD with Leary as its chief spokesman. Ginsberg and Leary decided that a series of well-established literati, artists and musicians should be invited to try the drug as part of the research project. Such people would hopefully endorse it and give it wider publicity and respectability at the same time. They included abstract expressionists Willem de Koonig and Franz Kline, and bebop masters Dizzy Gillespie and Thelonius Monk. But top of the list was Ginsberg's old friend and fellow Beat, Jack Kerouac.

Kerouac had tried peyote long ago and mescaline more recently with fairly positive results, but by the 60s his life was seriously off kilter. The publication of *On the Road* had brought him the fame he desired, though that had only succeeded in adding further complications to a personal situation that was completely chaotic. His relationships with women had all gone wrong and he was now living with his mother, a stern reactionary controlling figure who dominated him and treated him like a little boy. She tried to stop him seeing Burroughs and Ginsberg, whom she regarded as degenerates, and even took to writing them abusive letters that, in the case of the latter, contained anti-Semitic sentiments. Kerouac led a kind of double life, on the one hand trying to satisfy his mother's demands and on the other trying to live up to his reputation as a Beat writer-hero. But he was coming apart and had descended into alcoholism, directing his massive energy towards marathon drinking binges of breathtaking excess and the inevitable bad behaviour that went with such drunkenness.

Kerouac was drunk before the psilocybin session with Ginsberg and Leary, and he jokingly baited Leary, challenging his 'psychedelic absolution' with the notion of 'Jesus Christ as saviour' whilst referring to Ginsberg as a 'Communist faggot'. As a result of Kerouac's antics, Leary had a rare bad trip and later concluded that Kerouac couldn't let go of his old-time Catholicism and embrace the tenets of the new age. Deeper into the trip, Kerouac too started to have a bad time, becoming paranoid and regressing back to his stay in a Navy psychiatric ward and subsequent discharge from the service. His final revelation was: 'Everybody is full of shit'.

However, after another series of crises, Kerouac was looking for an 'antidote' and he met Leary again, this time obtaining a dozen Psilocybe mexicana mushrooms from him, which he ate before accompanying Leary on a walk around the Lower East Side of New York. This trip was initially euphoric and Kerouac felt liberated from his current torments. But as is sometimes the case with psilocybin, too much clarity can become unbearable, and Kerouac had to face the truth that there was no 'new life' waiting for him around the next bend in the road – the message of his writing and the dream by which he'd coped with his vicissitudes. When Leary wanted to publish an experience report from Kerouac, he refused and reverted back to his familiar paranoid and hostile persona.

That persona carried over into Kerouac's current relationship with his one-time best friend and muse, Neal Cassady – the 'Dean Moriarty' of On the Road and 'Cody Pomeray' of numerous other Kerouac novels. Cassady had embraced the psychedelic revolution – he described psilocybin as 'the Rolls Royce of dope' – and in much the same way as he'd naturally slipped into the Beat circle in the 40s, he'd now teamed up with the next wave of madcap adventurers – Ken Kesey and his Merry Pranksters. Kesey had taken the place in Cassady's life that Kerouac once occupied, and unsurprisingly Kerouac felt sidelined and disdainful about Cassady in this new mode. Kerouac was now 'off the road', so to speak, but Cassady still wanted to be behind the wheel, his foot flat on the gas pedal, heading forever 'Furthur' in his role as the Pranksters' driver.

Cassady was now in early middle age, balding and a little ragged and wild-eyed from decades of amphetamine use, more recently compounded with LSD. But he was still as much of 'a character' as ever. In *The Electric Kool-Aid Acid Test*, Tom Wolfe discovers him 'in a kinetic trance', expertly juggling a sledge hammer and always talking: '…spinning off memories, metaphors, literary, Oriental, hip allusions, all punctuated by the unlikely expression, 'you understand –'.'

When the Pranksters came to New York, Cassady saw this as a great opportunity to introduce Kesey to Kerouac, and Kesey himself dearly wanted to meet the legend who'd penned *On the Road*. In their apartment the Pranksters were all high on dope and acid, and as was their tradition they'd draped American flags everywhere, and one was duly tied around Kerouac's neck. The reactionary Kerouac didn't like this gesture, considering it disrespectful, and he gave them a demonstration of how to fold the flag properly, his dejected mood obvious to all. He refused the offer of drugs, and when Kesey tried to cheer him up, he hardly reacted. The Pranksters' original footage in the film Magic Trip shows Kerouac sat alone on a sofa, sucking on a can of beer, looking glum and disengaged from the group activity. The get-together wasn't a success, and if anything it hardened Kerouac's contempt for the new 'acid generation'.

In a late novel, Vanity of Duluoz, Kerouac's eponymous narrator speaks of, '…those LSD heads in newspaper photographs who sit in parks gazing rapturously at the sky to show how high they are when they're only victims momentarily of a contraction of the blood vessels and nerves in the brain that causes the illusion of a closure (a closing-up) of outside necessities…' Kerouac stuck to the booze and it finally killed him in 1969, at the age of just forty-seven – but his immortality was already assured.

Again at Ginsberg's behest, Leary contacted Burroughs by letter, which led to a further fusion of the Beat and psychedelic milieus. Burroughs responded enthusiastically, saying his work had benefited measurably from the use of hallucinogens and agreeing to try psilocybin pills within the research project. But Burroughs' first experience was not a success – it nauseated him and gave him disturbing visions of green boys with purple fungoid gills. He had also been experimenting with DMT, injecting it like junk, saying the results were sometimes unpleasant but always interesting.

Shortly afterwards, in the summer of 1961, Leary brought psilocybin to a Beat gathering in Tangier that included Burroughs, Ginsberg and the writers Paul Bowles and Gregory Corso. Leary turned them all on with mostly positive results, but unfortunately Burroughs had another bad reaction. In *High Priest* Leary reported that Burroughs looked haggard and tense, almost collapsed against the wall, and he said, 'I would like to sound a word of warning. I'm not feeling too well. I was struck by juxtaposition of purple fire mushroomed from the Pain Banks. Urgent Warning. I think I'll stay here in shrivelling envelopes of larval flesh. [...] One of the nastiest cases ever processed by this department.'

Burroughs was in a weird psychic space at this time; his cut-up literary practices had given him a skewed vision of reality that affected his personal life and he saw conspiracy theories everywhere. Psilocybin, DMT, LSD and other laboratory psychedelics came to register on him as part of the problem rather than part of the solution. When he heard of CIA interest in the mind-controlling potential of acid, it only served to reinforce this viewpoint. Ultimately he favoured yagé and the ultra high-dose cannabis candy majoun.

However Burroughs did get to know Leary better, turning on again with him in London and then participating in the American Psychological Association symposium on psychedelic drugs in Manhattan. Talking with first-hand expertise, Burroughs outlined the diametric differences between drugs that had been lumped together in public consciousness as 'narcotics' – opiates, cocaine, Benzedrine, barbiturates and of course psychedelics, which were in a class of their own. Alan Watts and Gerald Heard also gave talks, and the conference was so well attended that people were standing ten-deep in the hallway and sprawling on the floor.

Burroughs then witnessed some of Leary's experiments at Harvard, and his reaction was most disapproving. Burroughs had expected a more scientific approach to psychedelic research, using sensory deprivation tanks and brain-wave monitors; but instead he found tripped-out encounter sessions, involving endless theorising about universal love, enlightenment and game theory. Afterwards Burroughs published an open letter denouncing the Harvard work, which left Leary mortified. Leary renamed him 'Billbad', and in High Priest he summarised Burroughs' accusation: 'Harvard's hallucinogenic drug monopolists cover travel arrangements but never pay the constituents they have betrayed and sold out. They offer love in slop buckets to cover retreat.[…] They steal, bottle and dole out addictive love in eye-droppers of increased awareness of unpleasant or dangerous symptoms.'

Burroughs' essential conservatism towards the psychedelic movement can be seen in part as generational. He was by then in his late forties, middle aged, and perhaps had lost some of his enthusiasm for the shock of the new. His brush with psychedelics was similar in trajectory to Kerouac's and also to that of another Leary subject, Arthur Koestler, who at the age of fifty-five found psilocybin an ordeal of rationality, offering 'pressure-cooker mysticism'. In 1979 when Burroughs was sixty-five, he journeyed to Switzerland and met Albert Hofmann, then seventy-three, and eighty-one-year-old R. Gordon Wasson – two other grand old men of psychedelia. They got on extremely well, with Burroughs most interested in Wasson's work on sacred mushroom use in antiquity and also in Hofmann's just completed book *LSD My Problem Child*, which Burroughs thought was a great title. All three of them were united in their condemnation of Leary and how he had lost control of the psychedelic project by sensationalising the experience. Such is the perspective of pipes and slippers!

So Ginsberg and Leary's projected merger of the Beat and psychedelic worlds didn't run smoothly, with two of the three major Beat figures ultimately failing to come onside. But nonetheless the interaction and cross-fertilisation that did take place was most fruitful, with Beat philosophy giving the new movement a strong sense of direction. Leary's book *High Priest* is in part a quasi-Beat piece of creative writing, with florid free-associative trip accounts and poetic non-linear mystical ramblings. Ever the chameleon, Leary mimics or 'samples' the writers he tripped with, so the Ginsberg chapter is like Leary doing 'Howl' and the Burroughs chapter like Leary's *Naked Lunch* and *Soft Machine*. Though Leary was deeply hurt by Burroughs' reaction, he continued to admire him as a figure and their friendship was eventually repaired.

If Kerouac and Burroughs remained somewhat bit-part players as the 60s cultural revolution went into full swing, Ginsberg progressively positioned himself centre stage, becoming one of its major movers and shakers, and an ambassador for Beat-mysticism to all, including the most famous. He rubbed shoulders with the Beatles, the Stones, Bob Dylan and the Byrds whist keeping up close involvement with Cassady, Kesey and Leary, helping gather support after Leary's 1965 drugs bust. Ginsberg was also very actively political, campaigning for marijuana legalisation and taking up anti-capitalist and anti-war stances – a hot issue as the Vietnam conflict escalated. Along with Kesey and the Pranksters, he was instrumental in diffusing a potentially violent confrontation between so-called Communist Vietnam protesters and a chapter of the Hell's Angels, who were

American patriots. They also turned the Angels onto acid. Tom Wolfe captures a snapshot of Ginsberg at this time in *The Electric Kool-Aid Acid Test*:

'Then Allen Ginsberg was in front of the microphone with finger cymbals on each hand, dancing around with a beard down to his belly and chanting Hindu chants into the microphone booming out over California, U.S.A., Hare Krishna hare krishna […] He was a lot of things the Angels hated, a Jew, an intellectual, a New Yorker, but he was too much, the greatest straightest unstraight guy they ever met.'

That image of Ginsberg was enshrined in world consciousness after he appeared at the 1967 Human Be-In in San Francisco, along with Leary, fellow Beat poet Gary Snyder – hero of Kerouac's novel The Dharma Bums – plus the Grateful Dead, Jefferson Airplane and an audience of thirty thousand. The media turned photos and cartoons of Ginsberg into emblems for the hippy movement, and he gained the distinction of becoming the one poet of which most everybody had heard, though far fewer actually read his work.

Though Burroughs wasn't anything like as publicly active as Ginsberg, he nevertheless also became an icon of the 60s era. He too knew the Beatles and the Stones, and through his friendship with Paul McCartney he became immortalised as one of the figures on the Sgt. Pepper's album cover, montaged next to Marylyn Monroe and below Fred Astaire. In fact Burroughs' influence on the music scene was as profound as his influence on literature. He introduced David Bowie to the cut-up technique, gave names to bands such as Steely Dan and Soft Machine, and became an inspiration and godfather figure to Iggy Pop, Patti Smith, Kurt Cobain and even Duran Duran! If Ginsberg's fame peaked in the late 60, Burroughs' was more of a slow burn, consolidating through the 70s and 80s, when he was back living in America, and reaching a high in the 90s, partly due to David Cronenberg's wacky take on *Naked Lunch*, which made Burroughs, now a gnarled old man, into a 'King of Weird' for a new generation.

So the legacy of the Beats extended through the psychedelic era and beyond, and all their books, apart from obscure publications, are still in print and widely read. Kerouac's early death only served to make him more of a legend, and his seductive weave of fact and fiction, mythologizing his famous friends before they became so, created a feedback loop of endless fascination. Much continues to be written about them and recent feature films have dramatised Beat life, such as *On the Road*, *Howl* and *Kill Your Darlings*. The pertinence of their activities and writings to today's alternative scene is as strong as ever.

CHAPTER 5

No Imperfection in the Budded Mountain
Allen Ginsberg and the Writing of Wales Visitation

by Andy Roberts

As an historian of LSD culture in Britain, I can honestly say I haven't come across much LSD poetry. Verse written under the influence of, inspired by, or about LSD is uncommon and when it does exist it is often doggerel, of the you-had-to-be-there kind. There are exceptions, of which doomed Brit Beatnik Harry Fainlight's *The Spider*, about a bad trip, is possibly the most famous. Another excellent example, which accurately and succinctly distils the acid experience, is Roger McGough's dry, witty 1967 koan-like *Poem for National LSD Week*:

> *Mind, how you go*[1]

At the other end of the spectrum is Lancashire poet and former acid dealer Dave Cunliffe's lengthy and descriptive *The Two-Hour Assassination of God*, the first and last stanzas of which are:

> *At 4am, she entered the brain of God*
> *And stumbled blindly through its convoluted*
> *Swamps until reaching a clearing*
> *In which was reflected the image of everything*
> *That had ever happened*
> *To anyone anywhere in time and space*

> *At 6 am she clearly and directly saw*
> *A myriad living things manifest*
> *In joy and liberation upon the surface*
> *Of a world which didn't really change*
> *Except some skin and scales just dropped away*[2]

I know. We've all been there!

Fainlight, McGough and Cunliffe's efforts notwithstanding, the fact is that Britain has only ever produced one *really* great and perceptive LSD poem. And it took the American beat poet, Allen Ginsberg, to create it.

Ginsberg, love or loathe him, was a major influence on the literature and lifestyles of the beat and psychedelic scenes. His story is largely an American one but he visited the UK on several notable occasions, including giving a reading on the same bill as Harry Fainlight at the 1966 *Wholly Communion* event at the Royal Albert Hall. His most notorious poem, *Howl*, a word jazz paean to a generation redefined how poets from the 1950s onwards wrote.

And Ginsberg liked getting high. Besides experiences with alcohol, marijuana, mescaline, peyote, yage, nitrous oxide, psilocybin, heroin and other mind altering substances, by the mid-60s Ginsberg was a veteran acid head, having taken it first in 1959 at the Mental Research Institute in California's Palo Alto.

The set and setting for Ginsberg's first trip were odd, to say the least. As Hofmann's potion suffused his being, Ginsberg lay in a windowless room full of medical equipment, listening to Wagner's *Tristan and Isolde* while undergoing a battery of psychological tests. He survived the ordeal, and passed the acid test before it had been invented, commenting, 'It was astounding [I] saw a vision of that part of my consciousness which seemed to be permanent and transcendent and identical with the origin of the universe... this drug seems to automatically produce a mystical experience. Science is getting very hip[3]'.

Indeed, he was so impressed with LSD he concluded it to be more powerful, more meaningful, than mescaline or peyote and so safe he even wrote to his father, encouraging him to try it! The experience stimulated him to write the unambiguously titled *Lysergic Acid* which opens:

> *It is a multiple million eyed monster*
> *it is hidden in all its elephants and selves*
> *it hummeth in the electric typewriter*
> *it is electricity connected to itself, if it hath wires*
> *it is a vast Spiderweb*
> *and I am on the last millionth infinite tentacle of the spiderweb, a worrier*
> *lost, separated, a worm, a thought, a self*
> *I Allen Ginsberg a separate consciousness*
> *I who want to be God...*

Ginsberg took to LSD, rapidly becoming something of a psychedelic evangelist. In November 1966 he suggested to a room full of Unitarian ministers in Boston, Massachusetts: 'Everybody who hears my voice try the chemical LSD at least once... Then I prophecy we will all have seen some ray of glory or vastness beyond our conditioned social selves, beyond our government, beyond America even, that will unite us into a peaceful community[4]'.

Ginsberg first visited Britain in 1965, appearing in D. A. Pennebaker's film document of the Bob Dylan tour, *Don't Look Back*, and in Peter White-head's film of the International Poetry Incarnation event at the Royal Albert Hall, *Wholly Communion*. He returned to London two years later in 1967, the so-called summer of love.

Infamous psychiatrist, R.D. Laing, and his friends in the Institute of Phenomological Studies (David Cooper, Joe Burke and Leon Redler) organised the ten day Dialectics of Liberation conference, to be held at the Roundhouse – London counterculture's iconic venue – between 15-30 July. Ostensibly about social injustice, yet ironically not featuring a single women speaker in its line up, the conference featured countercultural heavy-hitters including Stokely Carmichael, Gregory Bateson, Herbert Marcuse and Emmitt Grogan. Ginsberg planned to deliver a paper titled 'Consciousness and Practical Action'.

On confirming the invitation to speak Ginsberg contacted his UK pub-lisher Tom Maschler, asking if he could stay with him in London. Maschler was a high profile literary agent and publisher, noted in a *Guardian* profile as having 're-established Jonathan Cape as the blue chip literary imprint'. He was also one of the people responsible for creating the Booker prize.

A young Iain Sinclair, many years distant from his fame as novelist and psychogeographer was very much into film at the time. Sinclair was offered £2000 by a German TV company to make a film of Ginsberg's visit to London, filming him at the Dialectics of Liberation conference and in a variety of other settings, both in interview and giving readings. Ginsberg made many pronouncements about LSD use during the course of filming in London, and Sinclair's *Kodak Mantra Diaries* is an indispensable record of these and of the poet's London visit in general[5].

Following the conference, Ginsberg took a break from filming with Sinclair and was invited to spend the weekend at Tom Maschler's Welsh holiday cottage at Carney Farm on the slopes of the Black Mountains.

On Thursday, 28 July, Maschler drove Ginsberg the 150 miles or so to his Black Mountain retreat. After the pair had settled in at the cottage they ate and over dinner Ginsberg opened a small tin, showing Maschler two pills wrapped in cotton wool, saying, 'These are LSD. I thought you might like to try it.' Maschler was an LSD virgin, although he had often consid-ered taking it. 'If you don't want to, I won't either', continued Ginsberg, 'but you need not be nervous. If you take the pill I will wait to make sure you are OK before I follow you[6]'.

Maschler thought Ginsberg's 'degree of caring was seductive' and, considering the set, setting and companion to be as perfect as it would get, agreed to the strange invitation. Ginsberg, by now a frequent flyer, knew exactly how to handle a neophyte on the golden road to unlimited devotion and suggested they wait until the following morning, so the drug's effects would have worn off by evening and they would not be kept up all night.

Friday 29 July dawned, wet and humid in the Black Mountains, with cloud wreathing the surrounding hills. Pan had clearly heard the call and was marshalling his elemental forces in order to give Maschler and Ginsberg a day to remember. Maschler took the LSD and, once Ginsberg was certain everything was ok, he swallowed the other pill. In the early stages of the trip, Maschler experienced the usual strong visual disturbances, 'I took the pill and looked out of my sitting room window on to the mountainside opposite. The mountain gradually turned a reddish-brown and the earth began to run down the hillside like lava[7]'. After three or four hours, possibly at the peak of the trip, Ginsberg wisely suggested they go for a walk, no doubt on the principle that venturing into the great outdoors is one of the best things you can do with a neophyte tripper.

Both men donned wet weather gear and wellingtons and set off up the hillside to the rear of Maschler's cottage, into the great mystery. Maschler was somewhat nervous about the climb. In fact it is neither particularly steep nor dangerous but the amplified sensations of LSD could well have made it appear so. To allay his fears Ginsberg taught Maschler a calming mantra:

Um, Um Sa Ra Wah, Buddha, Da Keen E Eye, Ben Za, Wan Niye, Ben Za, Be Ro, Za Ni Ye Um, Um Um, Pey Pey Pey So Ha

Despite being high Maschler had the presence of mind to take a camera with him on their lysergic adventure. He took several photographs of Ginsberg communing with nature on the Welsh mountainside; 'the poet in his gumshoes communing with a chunk of nature[8]'. Maschler recalled, 'The hills surrounding my cottage are dotted with sheep and Allen saw us as just two more sheep under the sky.' Away from his home country, the city, the literary establishment, the politics and the weight of his own fame, Ginsberg's trip thoroughly embraced the environment. Maschler remarked, 'He was immensely moved by the landscape and in the afternoon, still heavily under the influence of the drug, he began to write a poem called *Wales Visitation[9]'*.

Ginsberg's hand-written first draft is reproduced in the 1968 Cape Golliard edition, the poem at the time of writing apparently have no title other than the date, *Wales 1967 July 29 Saturday*. The astute reader will note that 29 July was in fact Friday and the confusion of dates may have come from the fact Ginsberg was writing as Friday slipped into Saturday or just because Ginsberg got the date or day wrong! The beginning of the first, as yet untitled, draft of the poem is reproduced here, with spelling and grammar exactly as Ginsberg wrote them on that misty mountain day forty six years ago:

Thru the thick wall'd window on vale Browed
White fog afloat
Trees moving in rivers of wind
The clouds arise
As on a wave, gigantic eddy lifting mist
Above teeming ferns exquisitely swayed
By one gentle motion vast as the long green crag
Glimpsed thru mullioned windows in the valley raine
Bardid, O Self, visitacion, Tell naught
But what was seen by one man
In a vale in Albion, of the folk, of Lambs,
Of the satanic thistle that raises its horned symmetry
Flowering with sister grass & flowret's visible
Pink and tiny invisible-small
Budded triple-petalled bloomlets
Equally angelic as lightbulbs,
Remember your day 150 miles from London's
Symmetrical throned Tower & network
Of TV pictures flashing bearded your Self,
Link the lambs of the tree-nooked hillside of
This day
With the cry of Blake and the silent thought of
Wordsworth in his Eld stillness[10] –

Maschler and Ginsberg drove back to London, Maschler still feeling the psychedelic effects of his back-to-nature acid experience, 'On the way back to London I had a sense of driving over the earth, the earth that was underneath the tarmac of the road'[11]. Once in the city Ginsberg continued to hone the poem as he resumed filming with Iain Sinclair who noted, 'He's just been down to Wales, to the countryside, the hills. And has written (is writing) Wales - A Visitation.... He has drunk of the Black Mountains and is easier for it, is calm and reflective[12]'.

Ginsberg later wrote of the poem, 'Wales Visitation was written on the sixth or so hour of an acid trip in Wales at the house of my English publisher. The word "visitation" comes from the peregrinations of the Welsh bards, who went once from village to village rhyming their news and gossip. The poem uses two thirds of the notes made at that time, stitched together later.' In London, as the poem developed, it was later annotated 'July 29, 1967 (LSD) August 3, 1967 (London[13])'. Justly proud of the poem and of how he had captured his psychedelic ramble Ginsberg wrote:

> *I was interested in making an artwork comprehensible to people not high on acid, an artefact that could point others' attention to micro-scopic details of the scene. They wouldn't necessarily know the poem was written on acid, but with an extraordinarily magnified visionary appreciation of the vastness of the motif in its 'minute particulars' it might transfer the high consciousness of LSD to somebody with ordi-nary mind. By focusing the poem's eye outside of my thoughts onto external pictures, details of the phenomenal world, I was able to main-tain a centre and balance, continuing from beginning to end in an intelligible sequence, focusing on awareness of breath. It was coher-ent enough to publish in The New Yorker, whose editors eliminated the note about acid.[14]*

Wales Visitation is regarded by many as one of Ginsberg's best poems, haunted as it is by the observant ghosts of the English Romantic tradition, like William Blake and Wordsworth, 'Long-breath Blakean invocations[15]'. But as one of Ginsberg's fictionalised contemporaries (Japhy Ryder (Gary Snyder), in Kerouac's *Dharma Bums*) said elsewhere, 'comparisons are odious', and poetic analysis is not going to overly concern this writer. The poem's technical merits aside, *Wales Visitation* is, to me at least, a percep-tive description of what an acid trip can be like in such wild and numinous surroundings; the elemental qualities of landscape, plants, animals, wind, and rain, intensified and coloured by the drug's effects. Distance from his everyday reality as the counterculture's poet-in-residence allowed Gins-berg to drop his mask and just let the acid show him what was in the moment. As he later reflected, 'for the first time I was able to externalise my attention instead of dwelling on the inner images and symbols[16]'.

The poem begins as the LSD comes on, inside Maschler's cottage, with Ginsberg observing the weather and myriad subtle movements of the landscape through mullioned windows. He vows to *'Tell naught but what seen by one man in a vale of Albion,'* although his thoughts briefly flash back to the filming he did earlier in the week with Iain Sinclair, before the trip intensifies and he heads out onto the hillside. Then, a full-on lysergic celebration of and communion with nature takes place, inner and outer sensations mingling as, *'Roar of the mountain wind slow, sigh of the body/ One Being on the mountainside stirring gently/Exquisitely balanced from bird cry to lamb to this voice knowing.'*

As Ginsberg dreams the world alive, the symmetry of flowers suggests to him mudras, the bleatings of new born lamb sounds recall mantras. He wandered the hillside, Maschler following and snapping Ginsberg in a variety of poses; pensively surveying the valley, lying on the wet grass examining an incised stone, kneeling and gazing into the camera's eye. Aware, thinking, sentient. High. As the poem draws to a close he reflects on the fact that the experience had been about the minutiae of what Irish mythology refers to as 'The music of what happens' – '*What did I notice? Particulars!*'.

Ginsberg had clearly attained that most clichéd but no less valuable of altered states, the sensation of being at one with nature becoming, *'one giant being breathing-one giant being that we're all part of'*. The imagery of *Wales Visitation* was completely different to that of his first acid poem, *Lysergic Acid*, much softer and pastoral, concerned with observation of the minutiae of right here, right now, rather than the earlier poem's cosmic vision.

Back in London, the first draft of *Wales Visitation* written, Ginsberg's parents, Louis and Edith, joined him, and father and son (Louis being a well-known poet in his own right) gave a reading together at the Institute of Contemporary Arts in Dover Street on 22 August 1967. His freshly minted lysergically inspired nature poem under its full title of *Wales - Visitation July 29ᵗʰ 1967* had its first reading that night. The reading was recorded and later released on the Saga Psyche record label as *The Ginsbergs at the ICA*.

Iain Sinclair came across *Wales - A Visitation* by accident. During a visit to poet Nathaniel Tarn in Hampstead, Sinclair was given a copy of the glassine-covered Cape Golliard hardback, 'Reading it, I found out where Allen had been when he absented himself from the filming: back in my home territory, Wales, climbing the hills behind Llanthony Abbey. Doubling the metaphors of romanticism, a Worsdworthian high on a high ridge. Hallucinogenic tourism in the great tradition. With muddy wellington boots and a camera[17]'.

Wales Visitation was first published in 1968 by Cape Goliard Press (London), as a hardback book with illustrated dust jacket, outer glassine jacket and endpapers made of Japanese wood pulp paper. The text of the poem is printed opposite a facsimile reproduction of the heavily edited and corrected manuscript. The edition comprised 300 copies of which 100 were signed and numbered by Ginsberg and included a 45*rpm* recording of the poem attached to the inner rear cover.

A further 200 copies were issued by Cape Goliard Press. These were *hors commerce* (not for trade) and the edition was published in small, landscape format, pamphlet size, with card covers and endpapers of Japanese wood pulp paper. The last page was printed with 'An offering for a peaceful summer from Allen Ginsberg & Cape Goliard Press.' These editions have become collectors' items, selling for several hundred pounds.

On 3 September, 1968, Ginsberg appeared on the conservative US TV discussion show Firing Line, where host William F Buckley Jnr asks him if he has a poem and Ginsberg responds, 'An interesting project, which is a poem I wrote on LSD.' Buckley: 'Under the influence?'. Ginsberg responded, as he pulled out from behind his chair the text of Wales Visitation, 'Under the influence of LSD', noting it was 'a long poem, long enough to be entertaining'. As Ginsberg reads the title, Buckley interjects with 'w.h.?', presumably thinking, possibly trying for a laugh, that the title was *Whales Visitation*! Ginsberg corrects him and launches into the full poem, with Buckley somewhat inanely interjecting 'nice' after the first stanza. Ginsberg gives a spirited reading, complete with trademark stare and gesticulations. Across from him, Buckley's rictus grin never wavers throughout, but rather than the expected sarcastic put down, the best he can manage is, 'I kinda liked that[18]'.

Ginsberg revised and changed the text of *Wales Visitation* a number of times over the years, most notably on live versions, and the interested reader is urged to locate and compare as many as possible. A number of versions can be located on the internet, with the definitive printed version being available in *Allen Ginsberg: Selected Poems 1947-1995*. The poem is also on *Ah!*, CD 3 of the 4 CD box set *Holy Roll, Jelly Soul*[19], where a recording of the poem taken from The Richard Freeman Midnight Show is used, together with a backing track of Ginsberg himself on harmonium.

In March 2013 a media report announced that the part of the original typed manuscript of *Wales Visitation* was to be auctioned at Bonham's of London. Simon Roberts, books, maps and manuscripts specialist at the auction house said he expected the sixty-line, hand annotated, manuscript to fetch between £800 and £1000[20]. At the auction on 10 April the manuscript exceeded all expectations by selling for £3125. Ginsberg would have been most amused that the flimsy material evidence of his psychedelic intimacy with the elemental forces of the Welsh hills had been reduced to the mere exchange of money in one of capitalism's finest institutions!

CHAPTER 6

A Psychedelic Trickster

A Steve Abrams Obituary

by David Luke

I got to know Steve in 2006 after having seen his name down to speak at the LSD conference in Basel, Switzerland, to celebrate Albert Hofmann's 100th birthday. Steve was billed in the programme to give a talk on 'synchronicity and the problem of coincidence in the psychedelic experience.' I was just finishing up my PhD on parapsychology and luck at the time, and was doing survey research on psychedelics and extrasensory perception (ESP) on the side, so I had a yearning to hear what he had to say.

Steve's blurb on the conference website said that he intended to draw upon Jung and Whitehead, 'to resolve the contradiction between the ubiquity of meaningful coincidence and the paucity of experimental evidence for so-called psychic phenomena.' It also said he was based in the UK. This was a stroke of luck, as it happened, because I had been lamenting the lack of any serious academic interest in both psychedelics and ESP existing this far from California, circa 1967. Anyone who juggled Jung, LSD and 'ESP research at Oxford secretly funded by the CIA' in their bio had my attention. Unfortunately, I never made it to Basel for that conference, but then neither did Steve, but we finally met up at his place in Notting Hill, London, and he told me his story.

In 1957, while just starting out in academia as an undergraduate, aged 18, Stephen Abrams wrote a letter to C.G. Jung about his desire to use parapsychology to test the great psychologist's idea of synchronicity. Surprisingly, Abrams received an in-depth reply, initiating a communication that continued until Jung's death just a few years later.[1]

Abrams completed his psychology degree at the University of Chicago, his hometown, where he was president of the Parapsychology

Laboratory between 1957 and 1960. He began to work as a visiting research fellow during his summer breaks with the patriarch of parapsychology at that time, J.B. Rhine, at his famous laboratory at Duke University in North Carolina. Upon completing his degree, Abrams moved to the UK and became an advanced student at St. Catherine's College at Oxford University from 1960 to 1967. He headed a parapsychological laboratory at the university's Department of Biometry and, having some skill in hypnosis, he investigated extrasensory stimulation of conditioned reflexes in hypnotized subjects. He was also responsible for organising the first conference outside of the US of the American-based Parapsychological Association, at Oxford University in 1964.[2]

His PhD studies at Oxford were part-funded by the CIA via the Human Ecology Fund, a secret front organization for the CIA's classified MK-ULTRA mind control project. It was under the auspices of MK-ULTRA that the CIA funded numerous academic projects investigating LSD and other methods of altering consciousness, with the aim of finding truth serums and techniques for interrogation and brainwashing.

Abrams didn't know it at the time but, while embarking on his PhD, he was about to depart on a whirlwind ride to Kansas, via Alice's rabbit hole. Dr James Monroe, the executive secretary at the Human Ecology Fund (HEF), based in New York, had sent Abrams a letter in April 1961 saying that they were interested in assisting his ESP research at Oxford. Abrams, having no idea who HEF were, arranged to travel back to the US to meet with Monroe to discuss funding. Prior to leaving, he met with Arthur Koestler, the writer who would later leave almost his entire estate to establish a parapsychology research unit and chair at the University of Edinburgh. Koestler had given a talk in London for the Society for Psychical Research and invited Abrams along afterwards for dinner, along with the anthropologist Francis Huxley – (son of Sir Julian Huxley, and nephew of Aldous Huxley). Koestler was heading to America to attend a conference on mind control organized by another secret CIA front organization, called the Joshua Macy Foundation – although he probably didn't know it at the time because the CIA were operating at a very underground level. Abrams suggested that Koestler go to Duke University to visit his old mentor J.B. Rhine at his parapsychology lab, and Huxley suggested that Koestler should also go and see Timothy Leary at Harvard.

Taking the slow route home, Abrams sailed to New York and met with James Monroe and Preston Abbot, the programme director of HEF. Following a seemingly successful meeting with his new potential funders, he caught a flight to Duke University to see Rhine, and changed planes in Washington. 'Just for a laugh' he tried calling the CIA via the operator and asked to speak to the director regarding recent communications he had had with the Russian parapsychologist, Leonid Vassiliev – the first cold war Russian to communicate across the iron curtain about ESP research. He was told that someone would come to meet him at the airport within the hour. Abrams was met by the MK-ULTRA second-in-command, Robert Lashbrook, and discussed his Soviet link up.

Having called the CIA so soon after his meeting with HEF executives, the CIA did a security check on Abrams at Duke University. Abrams later reasoned that they must have thought that he was either 'telepathic or taking the piss' because the link between HEF and the CIA was a very deep national secret at that time. Abrams later discovered, through freedom of information access years later, that he had been given security clearance concerning his knowledge of the link, which seemed to be better than what must have been a fairly grisly alternative. Their security check would also have discovered that Abrams was about to take psilocybin with Rhine any day, and must have put them in mind of the CIA's earlier project, code-named ARTICHOKE, a forerunner of MK-ULTRA that aimed, as part of its mind control remit, to discover drugs which could be used to develop telepathy and clairvoyance.[3] ARTICHOKE had sent agents to Mexico with R.G. Wasson in 1952 while on one of his seminal trips to discover the Psilocybe mushroom cult among the Mazatecs[4]. Many years later, in an interview with David Black, Abrams looked back upon his unwitting intuitive manoeuvres and declared that, 'I was rather in a position where I could write my own ticket. I was asking the spooks to give me money to study spooks. And to overcome their reserve I had to spook them[5]'.

Arriving at Rhine's lab, Abrams was invited to take part in a drug experiment the following day and signed a consent form. Koestler had taken up Huxley's suggestion and had been to see Leary at Harvard a week earlier, and the pair were flown down to Duke by Richard Alpert (Ram Dass) in his private plane. Leary had brought a bottle of psilocybin pills with him and along with Rhine and his research team everyone had got high, and even attempted some ESP experiments, although there was apparently way too much laughter for the tests to have been taken seriously.[6] Koestler had a bad trip and had 'lived through world war three'. Rhine, on the other hand, was quite inspired and kept Leary's bottle of pills for further research, although he had terminated the nascent psychedelic ESP project by the end of the year, despite an improvement in test scores[7] and not before Steve had his first trip.

Curiouser and curiouser, upon returning to the UK, Abrams found in his letterbox a funding cheque from HEF as well as a letter from Vasiliev offering copyright on a manuscript in Russian on his telepathy research, hoping that Abrams could get it published in English. Abrams wrote to Lashbrook at the CIA asking for help to get the book translated, but

Lashbrook, seeing that Abrams had security clearance, wrote back in January 1962 telling him not to write to the CIA because HEF would deal with it, by which point the penny must have truly dropped for Steve.

Later that year, the Human Ecology Fund programme director Preston Abbott arrived in the UK to meet with Steve and ask him how his ESP research was going. Abrams asked him about getting Vasiliev's manuscript translated but Abbott replied that it would cost too much. Surprised at this, Steve surmised that Abbott was not aware of the secret CIA relationship with HEF and so, deciding to have some fun, said, 'But, the agency said you'd be glad to do it'.[8] Abbott initially turned white, and then fumed, having previously turned down an invitation to work for the CIA he was not best pleased to find the agency were his paymasters after all. According to Abrams, 'He phoned long distance to Harold Wolff, the chair of the Human Ecology Foundation [Fund], and insisted that James Monroe – his superior – be fired on the spot, as he was.'[9] A massive reshuffle began at the Human Ecology Fund and most of the board of directors were replaced in a short time. In the late 1970s, Abrams met Abbott again in London and the former HEF director informed him that half of the organization's staff had had no idea that they were being run by the CIA.

After shooting himself spectacularly in the foot with the CIA funding, Abrams patched up his finances with grants from more legitimate funders to continue his PhD research, such as the Perrott Scholarship, a bequest administered by Trinity College Cambridge, set up to fund psychical research (i.e. ESP). But Abrams was never awarded the qualification, even though he submitted a worthy thesis and sat his viva voce in 1967, largely because he had by then become one of UK's leading drug law reform activists and had organised a number of demonstrations and other actions with Oxford students during the sixties, which had embarrassed the university.

Having just formed SOMA, the Society of Mental Awareness, Abrams wrote an essay on 'The Oxford scene and the law' that was covered by the student newspaper and which claimed that cannabis users were treated more harshly than heroin users by the law, because heroin addiction was still considered a medical problem at that time. In January 1967, The People newspaper got hold of the story and emphasized the claim that 500 Oxford students were using cannabis. The Senior Proctor at Oxford had claimed that about 30 people were using dope and that they were all nervous wrecks. In response, and on behalf of the one Oxford student being prosecuted for weed, a lively ensemble of about 500 students marched through Oxford in protest of the cannabis laws. The story escalated and in February the University Student Health Committee heard evidence from Abrams who argued that the Home Secretary should be pressed to set up an investigation, and the committee did just that. The Government responded positively in April by setting up the Wootton Committee to investigate hallucinogens, but not cannabis.

Things then continued to hot up in the press with Paul McCartney saying he had seen God on LSD, and with Mick Jagger and Keith Richards in court on cannabis and speed charges. Following the heavy sentencing of the two Stones at the end of June a number of angry protests, backed by SOMA, began in London, and the musicians were released immediately on bail. A massive legalize pot rally in Hyde Park was organized and presided over by Abrams, who had devised a plan to draw flack away from the Beatles' acid image and take the pressure off the Stones by placing a one-page advert in The Times stating that, 'The law against marijuana is immoral in principle and unworkable in practice.' The text of the advert was prepared by Abrams and was paid for secretly by the Beatles, who also signed it, as did Nobel Prize winner Francis Crick, and a number of MPs, leading medical experts and other notable public figures. The advert did its job and sparked a national debate, ultimately influencing the Wootton Committee to go beyond their initial remit and report on cannabis, stating that, 'The long asserted dangers of cannabis were exaggerated, and that the related law was socially damaging, if not unworkable.'[10]

By July 1968, the News of the World were regarding Steve as the UK's equivalent of Timothy Leary and ran a front page story with a maniacal image of Abrams stating that, 'This dangerous man must be stopped.' This had come about because Abrams had discovered a loophole in the law that enabled cannabis tincture to be prescribed freely even though cannabis in its ordinary state was illegal. Abrams had met with Bing Spear, the head of the Drug Inspectorate at the Home Office, who had thereafter made arrangements with the UN to increase the UK's meagre legal cannabis importation quota some 17-fold to 254 kilos. As a result, the organisation Abrams had founded, SOMA (which had Francis Crick, Francis Huxley and psychiatrist R.D. Laing as directors), was able to manufacture cannabis tincture for prescription by medical doctors that were SOMA members, such as the medic Sam Hutt (better known as the country musician Hank Wangford). SOMA were also researching alkaloids derived from cannabis, and investigated the use of pure THC, the main psychoactive chemical in cannabis. After some initial problems with the formula, which was corrected by Crick, SOMA's chief chemist Dick Pountain manufactured an experimental batch of seven grams of relatively pure THC at the cost of £1,600 – a considerable amount of money at the time. Abrams, as he delighted in telling me, smoked the whole thing over a weekend with his acquaintances and remarked that, 'It was like the very finest Moroccan kief with a hint of cocaine. It was very, very good dope'.

Listening to Steve's stories – all well evidenced – over the years I came to admire his association with what Jung identified as the *trickster archetype*. He was an exceptional and humorous intellect who could run rings around people, never suffered fools, and yet seemingly always remained honest and compassionate – no matter whom he was dealing with. He was also an exceptional raconteur and named the good and the great among his friends, be they leading musicians, politicians, scientists, psychiatrists, parapsychologists, activists or LSD-ring mastermind criminals on the run.

Perhaps my favourite story of Steve's concerned the occasion he and R.D. Laing were visited by detective inspector Richard Lee, the lead officer of Operation Julie – the UK's largest LSD bust that ended in the arrest of 130 people and put an end to a conspiracy that had produced over 100 million doses of acid in Britain over a six-year period. Because of their association with one of the ring leaders of the Brotherhood of Eternal Love – the world's biggest LSD manufacturers, busted in 1972 – the police had been interested in Abrams and the psychiatrist Laing, a leading figure in the anti-psychiatry movement who had pioneered the use of LSD therapy for schizophrenia. Through Bing Spear at the Home Office, Lee made arrangements to visit Laing and Abrams in 1977, shortly after the bust, for a 'social', and arrived at Laing's place with his driver. Informing them both that they were in the clear over Operation Julie, the four of them had a frank discussion, over copious whiskies, concerning psychiatry and the politics of LSD and cannabis. Lubricated by the scotch, Laing and Abrams were able to convince both officers of the folly of the drug laws and urged them both to quit the force, which, upon staggering back into work later that day, they both did, as did several other members of the Operation Julie team.[11]

Fast-forwarding to 2006, Steve never gave this talk at the Basel conference as he was unable to leave his house in Notting Hill, London, to make the trip, because he had emphysema. To my knowledge Steve never left the house from that point on as he had difficulty breathing, and was ultimately unable to breathe at all without a near continuous supplement of oxygen throughout the day. That is until he re-discovered cannabis tincture, and had it supplied by an underground dispensary in London, which, after only one dose, allowed him to come off oxygen for several hours a day. He continued with his own treatment against his doctor's wishes, and it afforded him a lot of relief. He had hoped to further investigate the benefits of cannabis tincture and aerosol as a vasodilator in the treatment of emphysema. Unfortunately, before he was able to take his research any further than mere personal assay, Steve died at his home in Notting Hill on 21 November, 2012, aged 74 (b. 15 July, 1938).

CHAPTER 7

Watts Ego

by Robert Dickins

> *Is the ego not the spirit at play?*
> *Is jealousy not the bind*
> *Of the conditions of the state?*
> *Be free your self-consciousness*
> *With LSD, but return to Earth*
> *With your ego present and free—*
> *With all the love and the light,*
> *And the insights you've seen,*
> *Love light the ego*
> *And in play you are free.*

Introduction

Not long ago, a little of that very precious commodity named time was presented to me by the Great Goddess Circumstance. I decided to re-read a book I hadn't opened in almost a decade: *The Fairy Faith in Celtic Countries* (1911) by Walter Yeeling Evans-Wentz. He was a researcher who came to have an important impact on psychedelia through his translations of Eastern scripture, particularly Tibetan. It was in light of this that a passage from his much earlier work *The Fairy Faith* struck me as particularly interesting:

> *The dream life in its higher ranges proves that our ego is not wholly embraced in self-consciousness, that the ego exceeds self-consciousness. Instead of a continuity of consciousness we have parallel states of consciousness for the one subject, the Ego*[1]

Drawing on the early theories of Sigmund Freud, in particular *The Interpretation of Dreams* (1901), Evans-Wentz postulated that the subject - ego - can experience a range of states of consciousness that exist in parallel with one another, for instance the ego experiences the dream state when 'self-consciousness' is put to one side. Self-consciousness, here, can be described as one's personal mode - a social identity with its particular desires, memories and socio-cultural constructs. The ego as subject, therefore, mediates these different states of consciousness. This is, of course, categorically not the limit of conscious experience according psychedelic discourse.

Fast-forward 50 years to the era of Psychedelia, and *The Psychedelic Experience* (TPE) by Timothy Leary, Ralph Metzner, and Richard Alpert, was being published as a guide book for trippers. The guide was based on *The Tibetan Book of the Dead*, edited by Evans-Wentz, and also included a dedication to *The Fairy Faith* author. A culturally important text in psychedelic literature, TPE is explicitly about employing psychedelic substances in order produce a state of ego-loss. In this sense, the ego is no longer the mediator of different states of consciousness but rather is a state of consciousness to be dissolved in itself.

Ego-loss is equated with a journey through death. The original Tibetan scripture was read over the dead and dying in order to guide them to a white light, whereupon, according to their tradition, they are liberated from reincarnation into another form of individualised consciousness and return instead to whence they came: the Void. TPE ascribes a similar mechanism so far as one is guided to the white light on LSD and experiences what they call 'ego death/dissolution'.

The psychedelic approach differs so far as if one experiences the white light, you still return to a prior individualized state thereafter. Thus ego is not the totality of subject; it represents a faction within it. If one understands TPE within a medical/therapeutic context, then the ego is both cause/symptom of a pathology - propagating a self-obsessed, illusory mental state (I/ego). One, according to other psychedelic works, that is perpetuated by certain Western value systems:

> *Use your foresight to choose a good post-session robot. Do not be attracted to your old ego. Whether you choose to pursue power, or status, or wisdom, or learning, or servitude, or whatever, choose impartially, without being attracted or repelled. Enter into the game existence with good grace, voluntarily and freely. Visualize it as a celestial mansion*[2]

TPE as a general guide book would have individual attachment to values transformed in people, and a new way of society ushered in.

The arc of psychedelic from medical theory to politically-charged cultural-value system is a typically complex story, and this article seeks only to contribute a single narrative-thread to the discussion. It will be partly told via an exposition of a nascent character in psychedelic literature: the ego. Still haunting the pages of psychedelic books today, the ego is characterized as both Scapegoat and Divine King, and in being so plays an ancient mythological role in the modern psychedelic narrative. For the purposes of this article, two writers will be considered, Aldous Huxley and, in particular, Alan Watts and his book *The Joyous Cosmology*. Both individuals partook of the early psychedelic experiments, and were among the most lucid of writers on the topic, both well versed in questions of the mind.

This story begins, however, with three spirits who encircled and partially possessed a new creation on planet Earth, one dutifully named *d-Lysergic acid diethylamide* (LSD).

The Possession of LSD

There are numerous ways in which the character of an object can be unveiled. In the case of LSD, so the story goes, it was in presentiment and accident that the action of LSD on the human body was first experienced. After earlier failing to pass through the bardo of animal testing, it was its efficacy in humans that underpinned its character, but just what that meant psychologically began life as 'phantasy'. Soon however, two spirits arose and quickly encircled and partially possessed LSD.

The oldest was Psykotomimetika. She was a source of experimental madness in her possessions. If LSD mimicked psychosis, it would thus elicit a pathological effect in humans, effectively a non-lethal poison to educate and examine. The experiencing subject, ego, would be possessed by the pathological manifestations of Psykotomimetika through LSD, and be temporarily maddened.

The second spirit to approach was the Son of Western Society, Psykolytika, who took the idea of pathology and embedded it in the society and the subject, and not LSD. The social neurotic is housed in the unconscious, a pathological side-effect from being 'civilised' creatures. Rather than disable the ego through being a servant of madness, Psykolytika served society, and wished to merely weaken the ego in order to treat the unconscious pathologies within. Psykolytika, partially undoing the work of Psykotomimetika by shifting the location of pathology, transformed LSD from poison to cure, but in doing so shared the madness around democratically.

In practice, under his guidance, low-doses of LSD serve as a therapeutic tool in psychodynamics by weakening the ego's defences and thereby allowing unconscious imagery to emerge encoded into the light of consciousness. Then the skilled servants of Psykolytika would analyse and treat the symptoms of our way of life, and thereby keep one's ego adjusted to society's demands. As a result, a struggle ensued between the two spirits over whether the chaos of madness or the order of society should be the governing principle of LSD's efficacy: the ego, merely the ancient Scapegoat in their play. Out of that struggle, however, a third spirit emerged that was both parent and child of the two.

God-fearing Psykedelika approached LSD, and s/he saw both heaven and hell, order and madness. Hir visionary eyes created an encompassing picture and was more powerful than the other spirits, seemingly able to capture the totality of imagination from without by bringing about ego death. Moreover, whereas Psykolytika wished to only treat the personal symptom of social pathology, Psykedelika was an insurrectionist and wanted to treat the cause: society. In this sense, LSD not only revealed social pathology, it actively worked against it through the transformation of values. The ego would not be temporarily disabled, nor weakened and adjusted, it would be transcended, and the influence of social pathology would be cut, giving the opportunity for the ego to form values other than those that serve (in this case) Western society.

Hir acolytes typically employed a single, large-dose session of LSD, that allowed one to have a transpersonal experience; known by its negative as 'ego-loss'. According to them, Psykedelika demands the sacrifice of the Divine King for the tribe's universal renewal, and the ego is that figure to the social body. The ego is dead, long live the ego. In other words, the death of the ego caused by a properly guided psychedelic session with LSD could be therapeutic for individual and society alike, when the shaman-self regains their connection to the Divine.

Of course, the question of therapeutic value lies in what can be achieved in the ego-loss state—LSD itself does not proscribe a morality. It would be God-fearing Psykedelika's acolytes who would presume to question the morality of new and ancient conditions. Suffice to say, for a time at least, LSD would be possessed by the equally revolutionary and evangelical fervour of healing society in the mid-to-late sixties. While the influence of each of these spirits can be felt reverberating around the character of the ego throughout psychedelic literature, it is Psykedelika who will largely guide us here.

Ego the Junction of Heaven and Hell

Aldous Huxley's (1894-1963) literary work on mescaline helped define the parameters of psychedelic literature, if only by providing a point of departure for a slew of following texts. In *The Doors of Perception* (1954) he wrote the following of the ego: 'All that the conscious ego can do is to formulate wishes, which are then carried out by forces which it controls very little and understands not at all[3]'. He goes on to say that it can cause the body to fall ill through its behaviour, so it is also potentially pathological.

Under the influence of mescaline, however, his awareness was no longer 'centred' on the ego, 'For the moment that interfering neurotic who, in waking hours, tries to run the show was blessedly out of the way[4]'. In its place, he experienced being awash in a flood of extra sensory data. The reducing-valve model, which Henri Bergson first developed, postulated that brain filters focused consciousness on utility and biological necessity. The ego is bound in some manner with this filter level; indeed, it is earth bound, where 'For most of us, most of the time, the world of everyday experience seems rather dim and drab[5]'.

Huxley is a link between Psykotomimetika and Psykedelika, it is he who saw the potential for both the madness of hell and the visionary state of heaven. More decidedly, the ego moves from being a pathology caused by LSD, to being a symptom of a pathological society, and the link between ego and society became an increasingly important question for those possessed by Psykedelika.

What world, or society, did the ego inhabit? One, according to Huxley's *Culture and the Individual* (1963), that was experiencing militant nationalism, rapid population growth and technological advance - dangers, he writes, that also emerge alongside possibilities. He describes a 'psychological inertia' in society that needed to be energized, and 'in these oppressive times a little hope [*psychedelics*] is surely no unwelcome visitant[6]'. Although he is careful not to fully endorse the use of psychedelics as a cure for 'inertia', he certainly poses the possibility.

Just how Huxley might have understood the ego-society relationship, and more importantly for him, the ego's occasional psychedelic absence within it, is illustrated in his novel *Island* (1962). The utopia of Pala is a peaceful society based on a synthesis of particular Western sciences and Eastern mysticism, part of which include the ritual use of a fictional magic mushroom described as moksha-medicine. It is employed a number of times over one's life, usually to mark certain ages, such as the entrance into adulthood, mid-life crisis, and death,

Furthermore, the moksha-medicine is employed as part of a wider Buddhist spiritual practice that aimed at the liberation of the ego: for both the preparation for death, and for the development of good social practice that is derived from non-ego awareness (Self). The Palanese character Ranja says that with moksha-medicine one can 'catch a glimpse of the world as it looks to someone who has been liberated from his bondage to the ego[7]'. Implicitly, Huxley is saying that by actively working against the obsessional ego (as part of a wider spiritual practice) a more peaceful society is possible.

The island's unexploited natural resources, however, mean the energy hungry world outside had greedy eyes turned toward it. The external forces represent what one might call ego-society—attempting to forcibly dominate the non-ego society. It is a macrocosmic metaphor of the Self being ordinarily dominated by a socially-contingent ego. The protagonist Will Farnaby begins the novel as a secret representative of the oil industry, but slowly succumbs to the allure of the utopia, till finally he experiences the moksha-medicine at the finale—while simultaneously Pala is invaded.

Huxley places his faith in the liberation of the ego, personal transcendence, yet at the same time is giving a damning indictment of Western society. The ego, when not weakened by ego-loss practice, is a villain that is manipulated by society to the detriment of the individual, humanity and the planet. Its wishes are pandered to by society in order to repress the hero of the piece; Self. Having enslaved the Self through dominance of the ego, Western society retains its dangerous omnipotence. Fight it, Huxley appears to be saying, by destroying the centrality of your own ego, and thus society's control of you.

Huxley's ego-loss reading of the psychedelic experience is described as being useful when engaged as part of a wider spiritual practice. In the case of *Island*, there is a synthesis of the psychedelic and Buddhist approach to ego, wherein ego represents a block (or illusion) that ordinarily debars forms of (to use a term out place) gnosis. The question is, however, does the psychedelic experience invariably lead to a set of Buddhist principles and a well-adjusted ego, or does the Buddhist practice condition both ego and experience? And more intricately, is the psychedelic experience itself conditioned to ego-loss?

There is a double-edged sword here. What happens if one removes the intellectual and practical framework of Buddhism? Unanchored, the ego may not let go, or do so unguided, and one might experience Huxley's hell, and not heaven. It would seem, therefore, that the set and setting paradigm is, as ever, key (if inescapably obvious). The psychedelic experience must be managed to intentions and, to do so effectively, the interfering neurotic, the ego, must be out of the way. For the hero, Self, the society-ego is an obstacle, and its destruction is the Self's coming of age: an important ritual before embarking on its quest.

In this sense, Huxley's thoughts tie in with those of Dr. Timothy Leary, so far as psychedelics are conditioning agents: Not only could they decondition the ego from society's negative influence, but they could recondition it to values deemed to lead to a better society. In Huxley's case, Buddhism. The major difference with Leary was that he believed society should be conditioned *en masse*—however, they both understood Psykedelika to be revolutionary, so far as current social conditions should be over-turned and a new social hierarchy placed: LSD was a tool for social change, and the spirit of Psykedelika would usher in a new age.

Watts Ego

Soon, some acolytes began to sense that god-fearing Psykedelika was a temptress and a seducer: and was not a revolutionist, but instead an insurrectionist, whose power lay in rising up in consciousness and shattering layers of conception, and then dissipating. The revolutionist seeks to replace one's condition, the insurrectionist plays for a time at being deconditioned. When god-fearing Psykedelika takes away hir tricky, magic mirror, s/he is god-fearing no more, and as one writer believed, the message is received.

A West Coast acolyte of Psykedelika, Alan Watts was a renowned speaker and popular writer. He rapped his way through religion, philosophy and psychotherapy, with a close regard for the psychology of religion and Oriental spiritual practices. Not only was he an apt research subject due to his ability to communicate complex ideas simply and eloquently, which he did famously, he also conducted his own home-grown 'research'.

The Joyous Cosmology (1962) is a gem in the poor box of psychedelic writing. In it, Watts expounds his vision of the psychological action of psychedelics, their philosophical implications, and their potential for medical use. Standing within the great tradition of creative non-fiction, Watts distils his experiences with psilocybin, LSD, and mescaline, into a single, sublime, trip narrative.

For all of the book's richness, however, it will be two strands in particular that concerns this exposition: ego and play. The former will be explored in light of the psychedelic reading of the ego, i.e. ego-loss, and show how Watts has elaborated his psychospiritual description using the notion of identity, which entails an implicit critique of Western society; following this, there will a discussion on the therapeutic role of 'play', which explores the insurrectionary nature of Psykedelika as a practical tool to overcome 'alienation', and its relationship with the ego.

However, before looking at how Watts elaborates on the psychedelic experience, we should note that he does not prescribe this experience to all trippers: 'I do not mean to generalize,' he wrote. 'I am speaking only of what I have experienced for myself, and I wish to repeat that drugs of this kind are in no sense bottled and pre-digested wisdom[8]'. In other words, his psychedelic experiences are particular to his own intellectual make-up, part of his own particular 'set'.

This is interesting because although he elaborates a psychedelic discourse that is closely associated with other popularisers at the time, he chooses to say that it is a *particular* experience. While it might be levelled that there is some elitism going on here, i.e. only those of 'superior' intellect could have such mystical and/or philosophical realizations, I believe this is disingenuous. Rather, he knew that he shared certain beliefs and education with his peers, and that their language in describing the psychedelic experience might simply be shared; a subjective value. Watts, it would seem, believed that descriptive language is simply a convenient fiction - one that he uses to brilliant effect in *The Joyous Cosmology*.

> *I become curiously affectionate and intimate with all that seemed alien. In the features of everything foreign, threatening, terrifying, incomprehensible, and remote I begin to recognize myself. Yet this is a 'myself' which I seem to be remembering from long ago—not at all my empirical ego of yesterday, not my specious personality*[9]

Watts is drawing out the experience of an emotional journey under the influence of Psykedelika. Indeed, it is a classic spiritual and self-help trip from the isolated isle of ego-fear, where one is alienated, to a state of empathy, affection, and love. *The Joyous Cosmology* is, what we might call, classically psychedelic, so far as personal identity is taken to be identical with the ego: ego is personal identity, or what Evans-Wentz called self-consciousness, and overcoming its conditioning is the therapeutic aim.

For your typical psychiatrist/therapist this process is known as 'regression', but psychedelic theory challenges the mainstream rational and scientific ontology, which argues that the limits of regression are defined by personal consciousness. According to Huxley, Watts and alike, one's regression is into a 'mind-at-large' - to use Huxley here - an interconnected and ultimately universal consciousness, which pre-supposes the emergence of personal consciousness in humans. The ego, however, ordinarily perpetuates an illusory identity and disconnects our conscious experience from the universal; leaving us 'alienated'.

Watts talks about the 'defended defensiveness' of the ego, which alludes to the ego being a mass of defence mechanisms that, when faced with the action of LSD, attempts to defend its ordinarily defensive self from the realization of mind-at-large; defending against the shattering of its own illusion. In this manner, Psykedelika wishes to sacrifice the ego that has become socially gluttonous, and teach that one is not a separate part or isolated island, but in fact an interconnected whole. Accordingly, one cannot experience the interconnectedness of the universe and the white light as an ego or, more accurately, one cannot remain the same self-conscious identity if one uncovers what he calls 'true identity': here, ego and personal identity are thus equated.

As Watts' trip narrative proceeds, one returns to an 'immediate presence' where the unfolding moment is in fact an eternity, where the present is a universal gesture, an 'eternal now'. Ordinarily, in our ego state, Watts believes we 'have lost touch with our original identity, which is not the system of images but the great self-moving gesture of this as yet unremembered moment[10]'. Having first regressed into an expanded identity, the process of ego-loss, Watts then proceeds to know his identity as a lived experience of the present.

In the midst of his trip he calls his friends over to tell them, first that they're all perfect, and then:

Life is basically a gesture, but no one, no thing, is making it [...] There is simply no problem of life; it's completely purposeless play—exuberance which is its own end. Basically there is the gesture. Time, space and multiplicity are complications of it. There is no reason whatever to explain it, for explanations are just another form of complexity, a new manifestation of life on top of life, of gestures gesturing[11]

Having first come to remember one's self as Self, through a regression in consciousness to a source, one awakens in the present as that same said form of consciousness: a becoming, the gesture. If not for the presence of 'greater' forms of consciousness, then Evans-Wentz' much earlier descriptions of the ego would ring true. Namely, that the ego, as the experiencing subject, has shed self-consciousness, and would then dance with psychedelic-consciousness. Watts is much closer to meaning the same as Evans-Wentz than Huxley was with the Mind-at-Large. Watts was not uncovering a map of the mind, he was involved creatively with the territory, through the gesture. He writes much more in terms of actions, flows and intercourse, just as the ego of Evans-Wentz moves between and explores waking and dreaming.

However, the ego had a new character in the psychedelic narrative, the Divine King, and it is its central, sacrificial, role that ultimately divine's the ground of Psykedelika; without it, the technique of cultivating divinity is lost.

Taken literally, there is also a philosophical leap here that that which is experienced for a period on hallucinogens can be a universal truth. In contrast, as we've seen, Watts believes the psychedelic experience to be particular, it is not 'bottled and pre-digested wisdom'. He is bringing his own intellectual 'set' - Eastern mysticism - to bear on the experience. It is important, therefore, to look at the practical and therapeutic elements he elaborates on as being contingent to the psychedelic experience: what is the action rather than the revelation.

The psychedelic experience, according to Watts, can directly inform our everyday consciousness. The 'unified and timeless mode of perception 'caps' our ordinary way of thinking and acting in the practical world: it includes it without destroying it. But it also modifies it by making it clear that the function of practical action is to serve the abiding present rather than the ever-receding future, and the living organism rather than the mechanical system of state or the social order[12]'. Thus psychedelic consciousness, *play*, informs and 'modifies' our ordinary consciousness so that it's directed toward the present. In the case of the prior quote, he politicizes the experience by making it a method of resistance against mechanical state or social orders.

Watts believed the 'conscious will' is an interior, 'inner echo', of social demands along with the identity boundaries put upon us as we grow up. It is a 'socially-fabricated self' that he at other times calls 'ego' and 'by means of this fiction the child is taught to control himself and conform himself to the requirements of social life[13]'. Society and the familial, therefore, perpetuate the illusion, they actively work against 'reality' and this in turn creates a state of alienation that, for Watts, is a pathological state. Hallucinogens, therapeutically, free us from the constraints of our own 'alienated' ego, by directing our consciousness toward the present; mindfulness.

If our sanity is to be strong and flexible, there must be occasional periods for the expression of completely spontaneous movement—for dancing, singing, howling, babbling, jumping, groaning, wailing—in short, for following any motion to which the organism as a whole seems to be inclined[14]

'Play' is the therapeutic mode that is occasioned by psychedelics. Putting aside the question of the 'true identity' for one moment, play is defined by an absence of the constraints put upon the individual by the expectations and training of familial, social, and cultural influences. Unencumbered, one is theoretically able to more freely express oneself, as it gives one a perspective outside of the conditioned, social ego that Watts deemed 'alienated'; thus it has therapeutic and resistive qualities. Play is not simply a return to child-like existence, but becomes a experiential modality in adulthood, one that actively works against the effects of external, mechanical authority.

It is therefore possible to understand psychedelic substances, and the mode of play, as political tools in Watts' work. They actively work against the authority of social demands put upon the individual so far as their action, psychologically speaking, enables one to become free of that conditioning. By freeing the individual, even if only temporarily, psyche-delics could be understood as significant tools of anarchic philosophy. This is an important point: psychedelics potentially produce a psychological anarchy. Not the popular conception of mayhem and destruction, but the one of political philosophy that rejects top-down authority.

It is at this moment of anarchic insurrection and politicisation, how-ever, where the mirage of a contradiction may be found. With the modality 'play', Watts has described the experience of losing ego-identity, which would seem also to be the major mechanism for overcoming alienation in society. The moral and ontological imperative of the true identity, over the personal, however, sacrifices the ego, imbuing it with Divine authority—a new master. *The Ego: Servant of society's value order*, is replaced with *Ego: Servant of the psychospiritual order*. There is, arguably, no anarchic space therefore, as a top-down authority is merely shifted.

.However, the psychospiritual order, the gesture, is Watts' own mental metaphor - Psykedelika's mirrored seduction - and he is fully aware it is a particularity of experience, and not a universal principle. Watts does not go so far as to say identity is itself an ontological foundation, he talks in psychological terms. Thus the experiencing subject never shifts, only the identity that is dictated to it by set, setting, and dose.

Thus play, he would appear to believe, is Psykedelika the insurrection-ist at work in LSD; a modality defined by the absence of certain social and familial identity forms; indeed, it temporarily works against their moral value systems. The reconditioning, as it were, is representative of set and setting, and is about any intended applications (or seductions) within the psychedelic experience. It is therefore culturally-bound just as with per-sonal identity; while the experimental condition produced by the action of psychedelics, *i.e.* play, would appear to be the 'true identity' of Psykede-lika hirself.

Conclusion

In conclusion, identity resolves itself in set and setting. So no matter whether that identity is personal, social, planetary, or universal, it is indica-tive of the intention of both the user and, if applicable, their guide. The psychological territory for such a possible identity transition to take place, however, is located in the action of a psychedelic substance. The insur-rectionist, Psykedelika, enters into one's psyche as a catastrophe—a rapid onset of psychological discombobulation that removes certain identity codifiers.

The move of ego from experiencing subject to particular state-of-consciousness, therefore, is firstly achieved narratively through giving it certain identity boundaries, and then giving it a sacrificial role in order to outline and maintain certain psychospiritual and/or divine grounds. The result though is to simultaneously politicize the psychedelic experience, freeing it of certain governing social principles, but also to replace those principles through another set of religious/ideological principles. Through essence, the ego becomes a victim of ideology.

If one were to follow Evans-Wentz and retain the distinction between ego/experiencing subject and self-consciousness, the political and/or social freedoms of the individual can be governed in a different space, *i.e.* play, which does not have any particular ideological precepts. It is perhaps time to free the ego of its psycho-literary constraints in order to produce a more radical and creative vehicle for both exploration and expression; one that is not determined by top-down authority or value constraints. In this manner we can more effectively break down the illusory boundary between sociopolitical and psychospiritual life, and attempt territories anew.

CHAPTER 8

Psychedelic Research
Past, Present, and Future

by Stanislav Grof

The use of psychedelic substances can be traced back millennia to the dawn of human history. Since time immemorial, plant materials containing powerful consciousness-expanding compounds were used in many different parts of the world in various ritual and spiritual contexts to induce non-ordinary states of consciousness or, more specifically, an important subgroup of them, which I call 'holotropic'. These plants have played an important role in shamanic practice, aboriginal healing ceremonies, rites of passage, mysteries of death and rebirth, and various other spiritual traditions. The ancient and native cultures using psychedelic materials held them in great esteem and considered them to be sacraments, 'flesh of the gods'.

Human groups, with psychedelic plants at their disposal, took advantage of their entheogenic effects (entheogenic means literally 'awakening the divine within') and made them the principal vehicles of their ritual and spiritual life. The preparations made from these plants mediated experiential contact with the archetypal dimensions of reality - deities, mythological realms, power animals, and numinous forces and aspects of nature. Another important area where states induced by psychedelics played a crucial role was diagnosing and healing various disorders. Anthropological literature also contains many reports indicating that native cultures have used psychedelics for enhancement of intuition and extrasensory perception for a variety of divinatory, as well as practical purposes, such as finding lost persons and objects, obtaining information about people in remote locations, and following the movement of the game that these people hunted. In addition, psychedelic experiences served as important sources of artistic inspiration, providing ideas for rituals, paintings, sculptures, and songs.

In the history of Chinese medicine, reports about psychedelic substances can be traced back about 3,000 years. The legendary divine potion referred to as *haoma* in the ancient Persian *Zend Avesta* and as *soma* in the Indian *Vedas* was used by the Indo-Iranian tribes millennia ago. The mystical states of consciousness induced by soma were very likely the principal source of the Vedic and Hindu religion. Preparations from different varieties of hemp have been smoked and ingested under various names - *hashish, charas, bhang, ganja, kif, and marijuana* - in Asia, in Africa, and in the Caribbean area for recreation, pleasure, and during religious ceremonies. They represented an important sacrament for such diverse groups as the Indian Brahmans, certain orders of Sufis, ancient Scythians, and the Jamaican Rastafarians.

Ceremonial use of various psychedelic substances also has a long history in Central America. Highly effective mind-altering plants were well known in several Pre-Columbian Indian cultures - among the Aztecs, Mayans, and Olmecs. The most famous of these are the Mexican cactus peyote (*Anhalonium Lewinii*), the sacred mushroom *teonanacatl* (*Psilocybe mexicana*) and *ololiuqui,* or morning glory seeds (*Ipomoea violacea*). These materials have been used as sacraments until this day by several Mexican Indian tribes (Huichols, Mazatecs, Cora people, and others,) and by the Native American Church.

The famous South American yajé or ayahuasca is a decoction from a jungle liana (*Banisteriopsis caapi*) with other plant additives. The Amazonian area is also known for a variety of psychedelic snuffs like *Virola callophylla* and *Piptadenia peregrina*. Preparations from the bark of the shrub iboga (*Tabernanthe iboga*) have been used by African tribes in lower dosages as a stimulant during lion hunts and long canoe trips and in higher doses as a ritual sacrament. The above list represents only a small fraction of psychedelic compounds that have been used over many centuries in various countries of the world. The impact that the experiences encountered in these states had on the spiritual and cultural life of pre-industrial societies has been enormous.

The long history of ritual psychedelic plant use contrasts sharply with a relatively short history of scientific efforts to identify their psychoactive alkaloids, prepare them in a pure form, and study their effects. The first psychedelic substance that was synthetized in a chemically pure form and systematically explored under laboratory conditions was mescaline, the active alkaloid from the peyote cactus. Clinical experiments conducted with this substance in the first three decades of the twentieth century focused on the phenomenology of the mescaline experience and its interesting effects on artistic perception and creative expression[1,2]. Surprisingly, they did not reveal its therapeutic, heuristic, and entheogenic potential of this substance. Kurt Beringer, author of the influential book *Der Meskalinrausch* (Mescaline Inebriation) published in 1927, concluded that mescaline induced a toxic psychosis[3].

After these pioneering clinical experiments with mescaline, very little research was done in this fascinating problem area until Albert Hofmann's 1943 epoch-making accidental intoxication and serendipitous discovery of the psychedelic properties of d-lysergic acid diethylamide (LSD-25). After the publication of the first clinical paper on LSD by Walter A. Stoll in the late 1940s[4], this new semisynthetic ergot derivative, active in incredibly minute quantities of micrograms or gammas (millionths of a gram) became an overnight sensation in the world of science.

The discovery of LSD started what has been called a 'golden era of psychopharmacology.' During a relatively short period of time, the joint efforts of biochemists, pharmacologists, neurophysiologists, psychiatrists, and psychologists succeeded in laying the foundations of a new scientific discipline that can be referred to as a *pharmacology of consciousness*. The active substances from several remaining psychedelic plants were chemically identified and prepared in chemically pure form. Following the discovery of LSD's effects, Albert Hofmann identified the active principles of the sacred Mexican magic mushrooms, and that of ololiuqui, or morning glory seeds.

The armamentarium of psychedelic substances was further enriched by psychoactive derivatives of tryptamine - DMT (dimethyltryptamine), DET (diethyltryptamine), and DPT (dipropyltryptamine) - synthetized and studied by the Budapest group of chemists, headed by Stephen Szara. The active principle from the African shrub *Tabernanthe iboga*, ibogaine, and the pure alkaloid from ayahuasca's main ingredient *Banisteriopsis caapi*, known under the names harmaline, yageine, and telepathine had already been isolated and chemically identified earlier in the twentieth century. In the 1950s, a wide range of psychedelic alkaloids in pure form was available to researchers. It was now possible to study their properties in the laboratory and explore the phenomenology of their clinical effects and their therapeutic potential. The revolution triggered by Albert Hofmann's serendipitous discovery of LSD was underway.

During this exciting era, LSD remained the center of attention for researchers. Never before had a single substance held so much promise in such a wide variety of fields. For psychopharmacologists and neurophysiologists, the discovery of LSD meant the beginning of a golden era of research that could solve many puzzles concerning neuroreceptors, synaptic transmitters, chemical antagonisms, and the intricate biochemical interactions underlying cerebral processes.

Experimental psychiatrists saw LSD as a unique means for creating a laboratory model for naturally occurring functional, or endogenous, psychoses. They hoped that the 'experimental psychosis,' induced by miniscule dosages of this substance, could provide unparalleled insights into the nature of these mysterious disorders and open new avenues for their treatment. It was suddenly conceivable that the brain or other parts of the body could under certain circumstances produce small quantities of a substance with similar effects as LSD. This meant that disorders like schizophrenia would not be mental diseases, but metabolic aberrations that could be counteracted by specific chemical intervention. The promise of this research was nothing less that the fulfillment of the dream of biologically oriented clinicians, the Holy Grail of psychiatry - a test-tube cure for schizophrenia.

LSD was also highly recommended as an extraordinary, unconventional, teaching device that would make it possible for clinical psychiatrists, psychologists, medical students, and nurses to spend a few hours in a world similar to that of their patients and as a result of it to understand them better, be able to communicate with them more effectively, and hopefully be more successful in treating them. Thousands of mental health professionals took advantage of this unique opportunity. These experiments brought surprising and astonishing results. They not only provided deep insights into the world of psychiatric patients, but also revolutionized the understanding of the nature and dimensions of the human psyche and consciousness.

Many professionals involved in these experiments discovered that the current model, limiting the psyche to postnatal biography and the Freudian individual unconscious, was superficial and inadequate. My own new map of the psyche that emerged out of this research added two large transbiographical domains - the perinatal level, closely related to the memory of biological birth, and the transpersonal level, harboring the historical and archetypal domains of the collective unconscious as envisioned by C. G. Jung[5]. Early experiments with LSD also showed that the sources of emotional and psychosomatic disorders were not limited to traumatic memories from childhood and infancy, as traditional psychiatrists assumed, but that their roots reached much deeper into the psyche, into the perinatal and transpersonal regions[6]. This surprising revelation was accompanied by the discovery of new powerful therapeutic mechanisms operating on these deep levels of the psyche.

Using LSD as a catalyst, it became possible to extend the range of applicability of psychotherapy to categories of patients that previously had been difficult to reach - sexual deviants, alcoholics, narcotic drug addicts, and criminal recidivists[7]. Particularly valuable and promising were the early efforts to use LSD psychotherapy in the work with terminal cancer patients. Research on this population showed that LSD was able to relieve severe pain, often even in those patients who had not responded to medication with narcotics. In a large percentage of these patients, it was also possible to ease or even eliminate difficult emotional and psychosomatic symptoms, such as depression, general tension, and insomnia, alleviate the fear of death, increase the quality of their life during the remaining days, and positively transform the experience of dying[8,9,10].

For historians and critics of art, the LSD experiments provided extraordinary new insights into the psychology and psychopathology of art, particularly paintings and sculptures of various native, so-called 'primitive' cultures and psychiatric patients, as well as various modern movements, such as abstractionism, impressionism, cubism, surrealism, and fantastic realism[11]. For professional painters, who participated in LSD research, the psychedelic session often marked a radical change in their artistic expression. Their imagination became much richer, their colors more vivid, and their style considerably freer. They could also often reach into deep recesses of their unconscious psyche and tap archetypal sources of inspiration. On occasion, people who had never painted before were able to produce extraordinary pieces of art.

LSD experimentation also brought fascinating observations, which were of great interest to spiritual teachers and scholars of comparative religion. The mystical experiences frequently observed in LSD sessions offered a radically new understanding of a wide variety of phenomena from the spiritual domain, including shamanism, the rites of passage, the ancient mysteries of death and rebirth, the Eastern religions and philosophies, and the mystical traditions of the world[12-13].The fact that LSD and other psychedelic substances were able to trigger a broad range of spiritual experiences became the subject of heated scientific discussion. They revolved around the fascinating problem concerning the nature and value of this 'instant' or 'chemical mysticism[14]'. As Walter Pahnke demonstrated in his famous Good Friday experiment, mystical experiences induced by psychedelics are indistinguishable from those described in mystical literature[15]. This finding was recently confirmed by a meticulous study by researchers at Johns Hopkins University[16] and has important theoretical and legal implications.

Psychedelic research involving LSD, psilocybin, mescaline, and the tryptamine derivatives seemed to be well on its way to fulfill all the above promises and expectations when it was suddenly interrupted by the unsupervised mass experimentation of the youth generation in the USA and other Western countries. In the infamous Harvard affair, psychology professors Timothy Leary and Richard Alpert lost their academic posts and had to leave the school after their overeager proselytizing of LSD's promise. The ensuing repressive measures of administrative, legal, and political nature had very little effect on street use of LSD and other psychedelics, but they drastically terminated legitimate clinical research. However, while the problems associated with this development were blown out of proportion by sensation-hunting journalists, the possible risks were not the only reason why LSD and other psychedelics were rejected by the Euro-American mainstream culture. An important contributing factor was also the attitude of technological societies toward holotropic states of consciousness.

As I mentioned earlier, all ancient and pre-industrial societies held these states in high esteem, whether they were induced by psychedelic plants or some of the many powerful non-drug 'technologies of the sacred.' Members of these social groups had the opportunity to repeatedly experience holotropic states of consciousness during their lifetime in a variety of sacred contexts. By comparison, the industrial civilization has pathologized holotropic states, rejected or even outlawed the contexts and tools that can facilitate them, and developed effective means of suppressing them when they occur spontaneously, Because of the resulting naiveté and ignorance concerning holotropic states, Western culture was unprepared to accept and incorporate the extraordinary mind-altering properties and power of psychedelics.

The sudden emergence of the Dionysian element from the depths of the unconscious and the heights of the superconscious was too threatening for Euro-American society. In addition, the irrational and transrational nature of psychedelic experiences seriously challenged the very foundations of the materialistic worldview of Western science. The existence and nature of these experiences could not be explained in the context of mainstream theories and seriously undermined the metaphysical assumptions concerning the priority of matter over consciousness in Western culture. It also threatened the leading myth of the industrial world by showing that true fulfillment does not come from achievement of material goals but from a profound mystical experience.

It was not just the culture at large that was unprepared for the psychedelic experience; this was also true for the helping professions. For most psychiatrists and psychologists, psychotherapy meant disciplined face-to-face discussions or free-associating on the couch. The intense emotions and dramatic physical manifestations in psychedelic sessions appeared to them to be too close to what they were used to associate with psychopathology. It was hard for them to imagine that such states could be healing and transformative. As a result, they did not trust the reports about the extraordinary power of psychedelic psychotherapy coming from those colleagues who had enough courage to take the chances and do psychedelic therapy, or from their clients.

To complicate the situation further, many of the phenomena occurring in psychedelic sessions could not be understood within the context of theories dominating academic thinking. The possibility of reliving birth or episodes from embryonic life, obtaining accurate information about world history and mythology from the collective unconscious, experiencing archetypal realities and karmic memories, or perceiving remote events in out-of-body states, were simply too fantastic to be believable for an average professional. Yet those of us who had the chance to work with LSD and were willing to radically change our theoretical understanding of the psyche and practical strategy of therapy were able to see and appreciate the enormous potential of psychedelics, both as therapeutic tools and as substances of extraordinary heuristic value.

In one of my early books, I suggested that the potential significance of LSD and other psychedelics for psychiatry and psychology was comparable to the value the microscope has for biology and medicine or the telescope has for astronomy. My later experience with psychedelics only confirmed this initial impression. These substances function as unspecific amplifiers that increase the cathexis (energetic charge) associated with the deep unconscious contents of the psyche and make them available for conscious processing. This unique property of psychedelics makes it possible to study psychological undercurrents that govern our experiences and behaviors to a depth that cannot be matched by any other method and tool available in modern mainstream psychiatry and psychology. In addition, it offers unique opportunities for healing of emotional and psychosomatic disorders, for positive personality transformation, and consciousness evolution.

Naturally, the tools of this power carry with them greater risks than more conservative and far less effective tools currently accepted and used by mainstream psychiatry, such as verbal psychotherapy or tranquillizing medication. Clinical research has shown that these risks can be minimized by responsible use and careful control of the set and setting. The safety of psychedelic therapy when conducted in a clinical setting was demonstrated by Sidney Cohen's study based on information drawn from more than 25,000 psychedelic sessions. According to Cohen, LSD therapy appeared to be much safer than many other procedures that had been at one time or another routinely used in psychiatric treatment, such as electroshock therapy, insulin coma therapy, and psychosurgery[17]. However, legislators responding to unsupervised mass use of psychedelics did not get their information from scientific publications, but from the stories of sensation-hunting journalists. The legal and administrative sanctions against psychedelics did not deter lay experimentation, but they all but terminated legitimate scientific research of these substances.

For those of us who had the privilege to explore and experience the extraordinary potential of psychedelics, this was a tragic loss for psychiatry, psychology, and psychotherapy. We felt that these unfortunate developments wasted what was probably the single most important opportunity in the history of these disciplines. Had it been possible to avoid the unnecessary mass hysteria and continue responsible research of psychedelics, they could have undoubtedly radically transformed the theory and practice of psychiatry. I believe that the observations from this research have the potential to initiate a revolution in the understanding of the human psyche and of consciousness comparable to the conceptual cataclysm that modern physicists experienced last century in relation to their theories concerning matter. This new knowledge could become an integral part of a comprehensive new scientific paradigm of the twenty-first century.

At present, when more than four decades have elapsed since official research with psychedelics was effectively terminated, I can attempt to evaluate the past history of these substances and glimpse into their future. After having personally conducted over the last fifty years more than four thousand psychedelic sessions, I have developed great awe and respect for these compounds and their enormous positive, as well as negative, potential. They are powerful tools and like any tool they can be used skillfully, ineptly, or destructively. The result will be critically dependent on the set and setting.

The question of whether LSD is a phenomenal medicine or a devil's drug makes as little sense as a similar question asked about the positive or negative potential of a knife. Naturally, we will get a very different report from a surgeon who bases his or her judgment on successful operations and from the police chief who investigates murders committed with knives. A housewife would see the knife primarily as a useful kitchen tool and an artist would employ it in carving wooden sculptures. It would make little sense to judge the usefulness and dangers of a knife by watching children who play with it without adequate maturity and skill. Similarly, the image of LSD will vary whether we focus on the results of responsible clinical or spiritual use, naive and careless mass self-experimentation of the young, or deliberately destructive experiments of the military.

Until it is clearly understood that the results of the administration of psychedelics are critically influenced by the factors of set and setting, there is no hope for rational decisions in regard to psychedelic drug policies. I firmly believe that psychedelics can be used in such a way that the benefits far outweigh the risks. This has been amply proven by millennia of safe ritual and spiritual use of psychedelics by generations of shamans, individual healers, and entire aboriginal cultures. However, the Western industrial civilization has so far abused nearly all its discoveries and there is not much hope that psychedelics will make an exception, unless we rise as a group to a higher level of consciousness and emotional maturity.

Whether or not psychedelics will return into psychiatry and will again become part of the therapeutic armamentarium is a complex problem and its solution will probably be determined not only by the results of scientific research, but also by a variety of political, legal, economic, and mass-psychological factors. However, I believe that Western society is at present much better equipped to accept and assimilate psychedelics than it was in the 1950s. At the time when psychiatrists and psychologists started to experiment with LSD, psychotherapy was limited to verbal exchanges between therapist and clients. Intense emotions and active behavior were referred to as 'acting-out' and were seen as violations of basic therapeutic rules. Psychedelic sessions were on the other side of the spectrum, evoking dramatic emotions, psychomotor excitement, and vivid perceptual changes. They thus seemed to be more like states that psychiatrists considered pathological and tried to suppress by all means than conditions to which one would attribute therapeutic potential. This was reflected in the terms 'hallucinogens,' 'delirogens,' 'psychotomimetics,' and 'experimental psychoses,' used initially for psychedelics and the states induced by them. In any case, psychedelic sessions more resembled scenes from anthropological movies about healing rituals of 'primitive' cultures and other aboriginal ceremonies than those expected in a psychiatrist's office.

In addition, many of the experiences and observations from psychedelic sessions seemed to seriously challenge the image of the human psyche and of the universe developed by Newtonian-Cartesian science and considered to be accurate and definitive descriptions of 'objective reality.' Psychedelic subjects reported experiential identification with other people, animals, and various aspects of nature, during which they gained access to new information about areas that they previously had no intellectual knowledge. The same was true about experiential excursions into the lives of their human and animal ancestors, as well as racial, collective, and karmic memories.

On occasion, this new information was drawn from experiences involving the reliving of biological birth and memories of prenatal life, encounters with archetypal beings, and visits to mythological realms of different cultures. In out-of-body experiences, experimental subjects were able to witness and accurately describe remote events occurring in locations that were outside the range of their senses. None of these happenings were considered possible in the context of traditional materialistic science, and yet, in psychedelic sessions, they were observed frequently. This naturally caused deep conceptual turmoil and confusion in the minds of conventionally trained experimenters. Under these circumstances, many professionals chose to shy away from this area to preserve their respectable scientific world-view and professional reputation, and to protect their common sense and sanity.

The last four decades have brought many revolutionary changes that have profoundly influenced the climate in the world of psychotherapy. Humanistic and transpersonal psychology have developed powerful experiential techniques that emphasize deep regression, direct expression of intense emotions, and bodywork leading to the release of physical energies. Among these new approaches to self-exploration are Gestalt practice, bioenergetics and other neo-Reichian methods, primal therapy, rebirthing, and holotropic breathwork. The inner experiences and outer manifestations, as well as therapeutic strategies, in these therapies bear a great similarity to those observed in psychedelic sessions. These non-drug therapeutic strategies involve not only a similar spectrum of experiences, but also comparable conceptual challenges. As a result, for therapists practicing along these lines, the introduction of psychedelics would represent the next logical step rather than a dramatic change in their practice.

Moreover, the Newtonian-Cartesian thinking in science, which in the 1960s enjoyed great authority and popularity, has been progressively undermined by astonishing developments in a variety of disciplines. This has happened to such an extent that an increasing number of scientists feel an urgent need for an entirely different world-view, a new scientific paradigm. Salient examples of this development are philosophical implications of quantum-relativistic physics[18]-[19], David Bohm's theory of holomovement[20], Karl Pribram's holographic theory of the brain[21], Ilya Prigogine's theory of dissipative structures[22], Rupert Sheldrake's theory of morphogenetic fields[23], and so on.

It is very encouraging to see that all these new developments that are in irreconcilable conflict with traditional science seem to be compatible with the findings of psychedelic research and with transpersonal psychology. This list would not be complete without mentioning the remarkable effort of Ken Wilber to create a comprehensive synthesis of a variety of scientific disciplines and perennial philosophy[24].

Even more encouraging than the changes in the general scientific climate is the emergence of a new generation of researchers, who have been able to obtain official permissions to start programs of psychedelic therapy, involving LSD, psilocybin, dimethyltryptamine (DMT), methylene-dioxymethamphetamine (MDMA), and ketamine. Thanks to the determination and persistence of Rick Doblin and the Multidisciplinary Association for Psychedelic Research (MAPS), we are now experiencing a remarkable global renaissance of psychedelic research.

In the United States, several major universities have returned to psychedelic research—Harvard University, University of California in Los Angeles (UCLA), the Johns Hopkins University, State University of New York (SUNY), University of California in San Francisco (UCSF), and University of Arizona (UA). Dr. Michael Mithoeffer and his wife Annie have reported positive results with the use of MDMA in the treatment of post-traumatic stress disorder; their work could have important implications for solving the formidable problem of emotional disturbances in war veterans. And important psychedelic research is currently being conducted in Switzerland, Germany, Spain, England, Holland, Israel, Brazil, Peru, and many other countries of the world.

I hope that this trend will continue and grow in the future and that these remarkable medicines and sacraments will eventually return into healing, spiritual, and ritual practice guided by responsible therapists, researchers, and spiritual groups. If this happens. psychedelics will regain the important role that they played in many ancient and native societies. This would fulfill the dream of Albert Hofmann, the father of LSD, who envisioned what he called 'New Eleusis,' a future society in which these extraordinary substances would be used for the benefit of individuals, as well as society as a whole.

CHAPTER 9

A Psychedelic Researcher

The pitfalls and pleasures campaigning for psychedelic research in the British medical profession, the media, and the general public

by Ben Sessa

I qualified in medicine from University College London in 1997, special-ised in mental health and now spend most of my time working as a child and adolescent psychiatrist in Bristol. But alongside my day job, for the last decade, I have also been involved in psychedelic medical research. I began this unusual career interest in 2005 with an article in the British Journal of Psychiatry in which I described the emerging re-visiting of research into drugs like LSD, Psilocybin, MDMA, Ketamine and Ibogaine as adjuncts to psychotherapy for the treatment of unremitting anxiety disorders. At that time there were few other people within UK medicine discussing this type of research – though plenty from the United States, other professions and the disparate tribes of recreational drug users.

Much to my surprise that first article was well received and it lead to a succession of invitations throughout the country to lecture at medical schools and hospitals, as well as questions from other psychiatrists inter-ested to learn more about this peculiar subject. More published papers fol-lowed in medical journals and in 2007 I joined David Nutt at the Psychopharmacology Unit at Bristol University as a research associate. Whilst there I took part in the newly emerging psilocybin studies with Robin Carhart-Harris; becoming the first person in the UK to be legally given a psychedelic drug in forty years when Professor Nutt, as part of our pilot study, injected me with 1.5mg of intravenous psilocybin.

I subsequently contributed a paper, for David Nutt, in favour of MDMA research to the now infamous ACMD review of Ecstasy commissioned by the government, which lead to David's unforgettable comments about horse riding and his eventual sacking from the government body he chaired. He left the department and moved to Imperial University London, where he now resides, and with ten times more scanners than they ever gave him to play with at Bristol University he is perfectly happy there.

Despite having such an idiosyncratic and poorly understood research interest I have found an overwhelming level of support from my non-psychedelic colleagues in the NHS. I am frequently awarded leave and funding to present on psychedelics nationally and internationally and am allowed a certain amount of free time within my NHS timetable to pursue this field of interest. I am deeply grateful for my colleagues and employers for such generosity. Especially as they often don't understand what it is I do with psychedelics. Nevertheless, perhaps they recognise that whilst I continue to get published in this field it is a worthwhile research trajectory, even though it is certainly on the fringe of mainstream medicine.

I have also had helpful and encouraging validation for this research topic coming from the Royal College of Psychiatrists and mainstream publications such as the Journal of Psychopharmacology and the Lancet. I have presented several symposia at College conferences, as well as fielding any relevant calls from the press that get directed towards the College. Unwittingly, it seems, I have become the psychiatric profession's 'voice of LSD and Ecstasy'.

Not that it has all been plain sailing. Along the way a number of less open-minded colleagues have not been so supportive. Some have told me my research is 'career suicide' and that the time and money could be better spent elsewhere. They have suggested I consider researching more wholesome topics such as antidepressants, antipsychotics or any of the other packaged products dished out to us psychiatrists by the pharmaceutical industry. However, I passionately disagree. Two-dozen peer-reviewed papers and annual international invitations to speak can hardly be seen as a waste of time. Furthermore, I published a text book – *The Psychedelic Renaissance* - for use by trainee doctors and the general public, bringing them up to date on the latest research in the field of psychedelic drugs. And by final way of validation, the Royal College commissioned me to write a teaching module on psychedelic research for their development and education service, which truly gives the stamp of approval that psychedelic medicine is a subject worthy of pursuit for career doctors.

So, in general, I feel the medical profession has accepted the growing re-emergence of psychedelic research with a reasonably warm attitude. Doctors are often rather conservative, cautious people, as well as being deeply concerned for their patients' welfare, so they are on guard against anything that could be of harm. In this respect it is understandable that they approach the psychedelic drugs with trepidation. However, they are also people with a keen eye on emerging evidence, so they are able to see through the media scare tactics – on the whole – and accept robust scientific data when it is available.

And this is what the modern world of psychedelic research is all about; a strict avoidance of the pseudo-scientific hyperbole and a rigorous search for hard data about the safety and efficacy of these marvelous medicines. I wish the same approach could be said of the general public.

Unfortunately the UK media remain unhelpfully wedded to the seduction of eye-catching headlines more than to the assiduous gathering of balanced data. Alongside my efforts to convince the medical profession of the value and benefits of psychedelic therapies I have been keen to use my position to inform the popular media in the same topic. But on several occasions I have become unstuck. One main issue is that non-scientists (such as newspaper editors) have a tendency to not compare like with like. In particular they may counter a perfectly reasonable scientific argument with a less rational emotional line of reasoning.

An example of this occurred when, six years ago, I spoke to a journalist about the value of MDMA Therapy. I was careful to present, as usual, a balanced and cautious approach, using scientific data and clinical evidence to support my arguments in favour of the research. But the journalist then took my interview to his boss, the newspaper editor, who, in an effort to 'create a balance' went on to interview the parents of a teenager who tragically died after taking ten ecstasy tablets in a nightclub. The paper then used this as a counter argument to my interview, under the headline 'British Doctor says Give Kids Ecstasy' (or something similarly ridiculous). I was furious. I rang the editor and said, 'At what point did I ever recommend anyone taking ten ecstasy tablets in a night club?' But I got nowhere. The emotional argument of grieving parents is a powerful force, and one that can trump any amount of scientific evidence – even if they are describing completely different issues. I learned an important lesson about the difference between the sensitive journalist – who genuinely wants the facts – and the ruthless editor, who writes the headlines and is thinking only of ways to attract readers to the article.

A number of years ago I was asked to take part in Channel Four's 'Drugs Live' programme about ecstasy. I was in communication with the show's producers for some months in advance and was party to the development of the script as it took shape. I was due to be on the show to talk about a new 'MDMA for PTSD' project that was being planned.

The week of the live broadcast I took two days away from my patients. Channel Four kindly put me up in a swanky hotel in Chelsea and I sat in the audience, according to the script, diligently waiting for the microphone to come my way so I could share my thoughts on the safe and efficacious value of clinical MDMA research. At every advert break throughout the show I was told: 'Stand by Dr Sessa! You're on next!' but Jon Snow never spoke to me about clinical MDMA.

Instead what I saw was the producers returning the presenters again and again back to repeated stories of 'the dangers of ecstasy', re-interviewing on multiple occasions a non-clinical professor of psychopharmacology and a collection of burned-out gurning ravers about their exploits in nightclubs taking recreational drugs.

Channel Four, who were anxious at possibly appearing 'soft on drugs', had pulled my appearance at the last minute because of a top-down decision. In order to 'present a balance' they overly crowded the programme with negative reporting at the cost of dropping the far more realistic issue of the safe use of clinical MDMA. It seems that after all these years neither Channel Four nor their anti-MDMA professor could entangle the difference between recreational ecstasy use and clinical MDMA.

The day after the final programme I was staggered to see that the professor in question had written to The Telegraph complaining that he felt he was not given adequate airtime to express his opinions on the programme! I wrote to the paper in reply and my letter was published, with the counter argument that he was given far too much exposure for his minority views, which were not representative of either the medical research community or the general public. And here is where the problem lies: a misunderstanding about how we manage risk in clinical medicine.

It is systemically flawed to look at poly-drug recreational 'ecstasy users' then describe minute, sub-clinical neurocognitive changes, and then compare this against the clinical use of MDMA in a controlled setting. I say sub-clinical because we know (those of us who work with patients and not just study participants in a lab) that despite 25 years of ecstasy use in the UK, with some 30 million doses of ecstasy taken recreationally every year, the levels of mortality and morbidity from this drug remains very low indeed. There have of course been some tragic high-profile deaths, which the media are always keen on reporting in stark contrast to the great many more everyday deaths from other drugs.

The truth is that deaths from ecstasy toxicity are very rare indeed. Rarer than, as we know from Nutt, horse riding. And so too are non-fatal psychiatric disorders. I challenge any psychiatrists reading this to tell me they see their wards and clinics full of the casualties of ecstasy use. Where is all this neurocognitive damage this Channel Four professor claims to have picked up with his microscope? In reality, after a quarter century of heavy ecstasy use in this country, the massive epidemic of casualties we were promised back in 1988 has simply not happened. Over ten years ago a department at Liverpool University that specialises in risk analysis was set up to look at the relative harms of ecstasy, but the project has since been shut down (they now explore gun crime instead), as it is now a well-known fact amongst scientists and politicians alike that Ecstasy is not, and never has been, a serious public health issue in the UK.

Perhaps the reason Channel Four failed to take into account the concept of risk-versus-benefit analysis is because it did not look at the problem from a clinical point of view? Everyday jobbing doctors know to weigh up the costs and benefits of the treatments we prescribe. We understand that no drug (or any other medical intervention) is 100% risk free. Whether considering something as invasive as cancer chemotherapy, or as benign as a sticking plaster, everything has a cost. In this context it is irrational to demonise the medicine MDMA just because the poorly controlled illegal use of ecstasy has some (very small) risks. This is a terrible example of medical practice and illustrates why non-clinical professors would not last a minute in a clinic setting if they are so rigidly expecting this fantastical 'zero cost' for their patients.

But the main reason why I, and the vast majority of the scientific and medical field object so strongly to Channel Four's risk aversive approach is that *recreational ecstasy does not equal clinical MDMA*! Endless studies on recreational ecstasy use are meaningless next to the proposed medical interventions myself and other colleagues are trying to introduce to the British public with our research on clinical MDMA. It is like reporting heroin abuse by junkies as justification for doctors not prescribing morphine in childbirth (though in fact much less so, as MDMA is no way near as toxic as the opiate drugs).

Perhaps I shouldn't be too hard on Drugs Live. After all, a programme on this topic even five years ago would have been 99% 'Killer Ecstasy' and, if you were lucky, 1% clinical MDMA. So the fact that they shifted this balance a little is, I suppose, progress. But my complaint remains that Channel Four felt obliged to strive for that artificial 50/50 equilibrium. In doing so they presented a clinically and scientifically unjustified argument that gave far too much airtime to the exaggerated risks of ecstasy and not nearly enough to the safe and efficacious research of clinical MDMA.

I doubt Channel Four's programme did much to convince kids in clubs to lay off their pills and powders – as evidenced by the tweets coming into Drug's Live that night, which (so the presenters told me afterwards in the bar) showed that the general public were overwhelmingly in support of hearing the positive message about MDMA, and not the silly antics of ravers and minority scare stories supporting a dated socio-politically motivated agenda.

So Channel Four certainly missed a trick that night in its attempt to debate this ethical issue. But we must not let the archaic irrationally biased argument against clinical MDMA continue to stand in the way of developing this medicine for the benefit of patients who may benefit from it. Like all psychedelic research, as I have discovered throughout my career with these fascinating compounds, the MDMA/ecstasy debate has always been controversial and fraught with ethical dilemmas. The quest ahead of us now is to insist that media and science alike stay true to the concepts of a dispassionate and accurate evidence base with which to approach the true risks and benefits of psychedelic drugs. To do anything less than that really would be unethical.

CHAPTER 10

MDMA: Wonderdrug?

by Chris Salway

Over the years a number of papers praising the therapeutic use of MDMA have been published and in this body of work there is some compelling evidence and argument. However, any potential negative effects of MDMA are given scant attention and dismissed as only problematic when taken in a recreational situation. There are very little or no concern that MDMA, used in a therapeutic setting, can be anything but positive.

In this paper I intend to describe some of the possible physical and psychological negative effects of taking MDMA. I recognise potential risks are less likely in the therapeutic setting than in the recreational, but they are present nonetheless. I will also discuss the idea that it is not possible to divorce the recreational use of MDMA and the therapeutic use of MDMA. I will argue that advocating MDMA as a therapeutic tool could imply that it is safe to use recreationally. This may not be right but, pragmatically, this is the way it would be interpreted by the popular media and the public at large. The final part of this paper will discuss ways in which any potential risks could be minimised in both therapeutic and recreational settings.

So let us take a journey through the brain and psyche after the ingestion of some MDMA and see what happens...

In the first instance let us assume that the substance having been taken is pure MDMA at a recommended dose of between 80mg and 125mg. Firstly I would like to discuss the effect on the hypothalamus. The hypothalamus is an area at the base of the brain involved with homeostasis; that is keeping everything in the body balanced including temperature control. MDMA affects the temperature control in the hypothalamus and users of MDMA will be very familiar with feeling hot after taking it. This effect can be compounded when used recreationally when, for example, dancing in a hot club. These 'thermal' effects of MDMA are described well by Parrott (MDMA and Temperature, a review article in Drugs and Alcohol Dependence).

I sometimes think that this is how MDMA works - to effect a period of cooking the brain which then leads to changes in the release of neurotransmitters. What can happen, not just due to the environment, although this will compound it, is that in some individuals (it may be difficult to predict who they may be) this can lead to a dangerously raised temperature – something called malignant hyperpyrexia, which is the situation if the temperature rises above 41° centigrade. At this point things can start to go horribly wrong, someone will stop sweating and if untreated this can lead to death.

Malignant hyperpyrexia is a recognised phenomenon after the administration of other drugs. It is a rare complication of general anaesthesia. The volatile anaesthetics – 'ethers' and the muscle paralysing drug Suxamethonium are both implicated. Doctors describe this as an idiosyncratic reaction meaning a highly individualized reaction to a particular drug. Certain idiosyncratic reactions are described with numerous types of drug and drug reactions. These reactions are very difficult to predict. In the case of general anaesthesia and malignant hyperpyrexia the anaesthetist would enquire of someone whether they, or their family, have previously had any problems with a general anaesthetic. If someone develops malignant hyperpyrexia after a general anaesthetic, treatment involves general cooling measures; stripping someone off, fans etc. Also, there is a particular drug called Dantrolene which can be given in this situation.

Malignant hyperpyrexia is implicated in the vast majority of MDMA related deaths. Any thermal effects of MDMA will be exacerbated by a hot environment, physical activity and large repeated doses. It is however possible that in a vulnerable individual, even with a pure dose in a calm setting, they can develop malignant hyperpyrexia. Cases of malignant hyperpyrexia associated with MDMA are very rare. Figures range between 10 and 30 deaths per year whilst annually millions of doses of MDMA are taken.

I have suggested that malignant hyperpyrexia can occur even with the therapeutic use of MDMA, however, it is likely that this would be even more rare than in the recreational setting. At the current levels of therapeutic MDMA use it may be many years before a case of malignant hyperpyrexia is seen in this setting.

MDMA can also have an effect on the pituitary gland, causing a rise in the levels of ADH (antidiuretic hormone). ADH acts on the kidneys to reduce urine output. If an individual then drinks excessive amounts of water this can lead to water intoxication, which in the worst case scenario can lead to brain swelling and death. This is another recognised cause of death in deaths associated with MDMA. All these effects of MDMA can be looked at as side effects or unwanted effects of the drug.

The wanted effects of MDMA are the increase in the release of neurotransmitters, serotonin and dopamine although, as I mentioned earlier, I postulated that perhaps it is the brain cooking effects of MDMA which then causes this release of serotonin and dopamine. It is the effect on these systems that are seen as the pleasurable, and some would say, transformative experiences of MDMA. Acutely, this can cause movement anomalies. This tends to be involuntary facial and sometimes limb movements. The colloquial term for this is 'gurning' and this resembles involuntary movements that occur in the long term use of antipsychotic drugs known as Tardive Dyskinesia.

So far in this paper, I have been discussing the adverse physical effects of MDMA. I would now like to discuss the potential for adverse effects on someone's mental health.

In vulnerable individuals it may precipitate psychosis and also mania. These effects would be worse in the recreational setting, compounded by the setting and dosage, but in the therapeutic setting they could also potentially cause problems. Dr Frederike Meckel Fischer in her LSD and MDMA assisted psychotherapy would exclude people with a history of psychosis and Bipolar Affective Disorder from treatment by these methods. A concern of mine is that someone, who has no history of major mental illness, may have an episode of psychosis or mania induced by MDMA nonetheless.

I would now like to move on to the subject of low mood precipitated by MDMA use. Users of MDMA describe a dip in their mood a day or two after taking MDMA referred to as 'blue Tuesday' or 'suicide Tuesday'. The theoretical rationale for this would be the depletion of serotonin after the MDMA induced release a day or two previously. There is no evidence that this can lead to long-term depression.

Now, I would like to discuss the MDMA experience in a less scientific or clinical way. For people first discovering MDMA they would frequently describe what a wonderful experience it is the first time they take it. Later ingestion of MDMA at other times is trying to recreate that first episode and is never quite as successful and this can involve people taking higher doses. The other thing I would say is that MDMA can be moreish. Some people will develop a pattern of taking MDMA at the weekend, feel low midweek, feel better again by the following week and then indulge again, this leading to deeper periods of low mood in between the weekend highs. As mentioned above there is no evidence that this leads to long term low mood problems. It can, however, have a very negative impact on several aspects of someone's life such as work, study and relationships.

I would argue that when someone uses powerful classic psychedelics such as DMT or psilocybin, people are unlikely to want to keep on repeating that experience. It is as if the MDMA takes you to the fluffy edge of this reality. It is a very pleasant moreish state to try to get back to whereas the more classic psychedelics maybe take one over the edge, a true alternate experience, something that can be very powerful and perhaps people won't be in a rush to go back there again. I would even go as far as saying that individuals who crave larger doses of MDMA are 'frustrated shamans' who some say should be taking high dose classic psychedelics. This brings me on to a quick mention of Ketamine.

What happened to the second summer of love? People have postulated that with MDMA getting harder to get hold of, coupled with an influx of Ketamine, that this leads people to switch to Ketamine. It may be more than that, although not a classic psychedelic Ketamine can give a more powerful experience than MDMA. It has been described as a near death experience, and the 'Near Death Experience' has been postulated as part of the classic psychedelic experience. Unfortunately Ketamine also has problems of moreishness and physically harmful effects. In this sense, these individuals would again be better off with the classic psychedelics.

Other substances, such as opiates and benzodiazepines, have been used by people to calm down the post MDMA edginess and promote sleep. I have seen people in my caseload, individuals who describe heavy recreational use, in quite a fried, depleted state as a result, which then led to the use of opiates and eventual opiate dependence.

I don't think it is possible, when discussing the risks of MDMA, to separate the therapeutic use from the recreational use. This is because, like it or not, whatever caveats are put in place, any medical uses of MDMA will be seen by drug users and the media as advocating MDMA use. I don't think the comparison of heroin applies. Heroin is used medicinally for suppressing pain and when used recreationally it is often to suppress emotional pain. Heroin use is not seen as a positive in these settings. Advocates of therapeutic MDMA use see it as a way of helping people to resolve painful past experiences. Recreational MDMA users might argue that if it's good enough for the doctors then it's good enough for them and they may have a point.

I would now like to look at what steps can be taken to try to reduce any potential risks with MDMA. Firstly, I would like to discuss this in the therapeutic setting and then go on to discuss this in the recreational setting. Many of the approaches are already employed in the therapeutic MDMA research that has already gone on. I am reiterating this and suggesting some other possible measures that could be put in place.

With a potential subject of MDMA assisted therapy, several points should be considered in the assessment process. Subjects should be asked about possible adverse reactions to any previous drugs, in particular anaesthetic agents and any family history of any reactions to anaesthetic agents. In effect we are considering malignant hyperpyrexia. Other important areas for attention are any psychiatric history, any previous history of psychosis or Bipolar Affective Disorder or a family history of Bipolar Affective Disorder. There should be some form of consent process whereby these identified possible risks, albeit very small, must be understood prior to consent. I would also suggest giving a test dose – a smaller dose of MDMA – to check if an idiosyncratic reaction occurs in the subject. It is not clear from the current evidence if this would identify people who could have an adverse reaction to MDMA but it would be a reasonable course of action.

Monitoring pulse, blood pressure and temperature throughout the procedure would seem excessive but keeping an eye on the temperature so that, if a very high temperature is developing, an urgent referral can be made. There should be some process already established for this; some liaison with a local general district hospital. There could be first aid measures in place such as fans and cool water to be used during the transfer of someone to hospital. I am not being alarmist or overstating the case, this may be necessary in one per 10,000 doses of MDMA, which is very rare, but with potentially very serious consequences.

As regards any psychiatric sequelae, a psychiatrist should be available whilst the MDMA treatment is being undertaken, post MDMA that night and the following day a review to ensure there has not been a development of any psychotic or manic symptoms seems necessary. Next, I would like to discuss harm reduction amongst recreational users of MDMA.

If MDMA were legal, there wouldn't be the attendant risk of unclear dosage or whether other substances have been cut with it. Failing this, the provision of a greater availability of testing kits to check the purity of MDMA would be recommended. The education of appropriate dosing of MDMA and education about potential risks (this is always a balancing act), awareness of risk however small without the introduction of paranoia is important. As well as educating potential users, it is important to educate medical services in particular A&E departments, especially about malignant hyperpyrexia.

With respect to the dip in mood that can occur 2 to 3 days post MDMA ingestion, it has been suggested that in the immediate days following the use of MDMA people eat Tryptophan containing foods or supplements. Tryptophan is the precursor of Serotonin and can therefore help restore depleted Serotonin levels.

I have tried to give a balanced view of any risks associated with MDMA use. I can see that it does have therapeutic potential but if this field is to progress it requires an open exploration of potential risks with measures put in place to minimise them.

CHAPTER 11

Trips to Sobriety

by Sam Gandy

The idea of ingesting a drug to combat addiction to another substance may seem strange to some, to others, heretical. There is however an ever growing body of research to back up the use of certain drugs for combating addiction, and the most promising of these are the psychedelics.

These substances are well suited to the task, in that they are have very low toxicity, are safe when administered in a therapeutic context, and are not addictive. If over used they have a tendency to induce bad trips, which acts as a buffer discouraging further heavy use. Addiction tends to centre on the denial or burial of past material, whereas psychedelics tend to bring life issues to the surface where it is hard to hide from them. They can also work in a multifaceted fashion on addiction, as shall be discussed.

Addiction is incredibly costly to society as a whole, with the National Institute on Drug Abuse stating it costs the US over $500 billion a year, with tobacco and alcohol being some of the leading causes of mortality the world over, and we currently lack any really effective treatments for either dependency. Thus it would be most unwise to pass up any potential avenues that may aid in combating addiction.

Ibogaine has generated particular interest for its anti-addiction properties. It is an alkaloid isolated from the root bark of *Tabernanthe iboga* which has a long history of use for healing and spiritual purposes in western Africa. A key part of its use in a traditional context is the death and rebirth experience of an initiatory flood dose, allowing the user to return to a new beginning. The addiction interrupting properties of ibogaine were discovered accidently by Howard Lotsof in 1962, who was addicted to heroin at the time. He was gifted some ibogaine by a chemist friend and when consumed he had an exhausting 32 hour trip. Going to bed likely swearing off ibogaine, he woke up the next morning surprised to find he had no desire to use heroin. This was unexpected and made a great impact on Lotsof, and although not a doctor or a scientist he campaigned hard for research to be conducted on its anti-addiction effect, and he played a key role in generating initial scientific and medical interest and research into the compound. Methadone is a standard treatment for heroin addiction, but this acts as a substitution, and is a highly addictive opiate itself, so one is simply swapping an illegal addiction for a pharmaceutical one. Ibogaine has a much deeper and broader effect on addiction.

Ibogaine appears to work on addiction in a number of interesting ways. The ibogaine molecule interacts with many different receptors in the brain, but has a low affinity for them. This is one of the reasons that the medical establishment is not attracted to conducting research on it; it is deemed to be a "dirty" drug, and medical science prefers drugs that are more direct and specific in their action. Ibogaine acts in a multifaceted way, even on a biochemical level. It works in part by resetting receptors in the brain to a pre-addiction state. It can alleviate the withdrawals from drugs such as opiates, which is a big help in breaking the addiction cycle. It also induces a waking dream state, a highly personable experience taking place behind closed eyelids, where one will likely encounter repressed memories and examine past and current life issues, but in an emotionally detached manner. This period of reflection aids in a detached introspective examination of the roots of one's addiction and the behaviour patterns associated with it. Ibogaine is converted to noribogaine by the liver and has prolonged effects, often experienced as an afterglow and mood lift post session, and this compound is thought to play a role in the anti-addictive effects of ibogaine.

Ibogaine also causes a long term increase in the expression of a growth factor protein known as the *glial cell line-derived neurotrophic factor* (GDNF). GDNF is a highly neuroprotective protein, promoting the survival and differentiation of dopaminergic and motor neurons, and has the ability to induce neuronal sprouting in the brain. GDNF also appears to play a major role in ibogaine's longer term anti-addiction effect. Ibogaine increases GDNF via an autoregulatory positive feedback loop. So the increase in GDNF caused by ibogaine induces neurons to produce mRNA, which acts as biochemical blueprint in the manufacture of further GDNF. Other lifestyle factors, such as exercise and sunlight, also increase expression of this protein. Ibogaine is highly lipophilic, and can remain in body tissues for months, so extending this anti-addiction effect. People have found booster doses following a flood session helpful in keeping on this path, and others have had success through microdosing, as the effects of ibogaine and its sister alkaloids in iboga are cumulative and build up in one's system over time. So for some this may be a beneficial and safe approach to using this plant in a way that can be integrated into day to day life and without the ordeal of a flood dose experience.

Ibogaine, the classic 'anti-drug drug' is not a panacea for treating addiction. It can however provide a window through which people that have the will can enact change. If seeking ibogaine in this context, the person seeking treatment will require support post session and changes in life style should be made prior, such as avoiding situations or people that may have associations of past drug use. Ibogaine requires work and will on behalf of the person using it to maximise chances of success. MAPS is conducting ongoing research at ibogaine clinics in New Zealand and Mexico looking at ibogaine's long term effects on addiction.

A structured and supportive setting plays a key role in addiction treatment, and this can take a number of different forms. In the Native American Church (NAC), peyote is viewed as a powerful treatment for alcoholism. Members of the Church believe peyote will show them the truth about their lives and give them insight and guidance, and past studies have found positive effects of peyote on social, mental and physical well-being. Suggestibility may also be playing a role in this setting. Alcoholism is a major affliction among the Native American population, around four times higher than the US average, and the NAC offers a chance to combat this.

In the UK alone, alcoholism costs the NHS £3 billion a year, and this figure is rising, with alcohol misuse being one of the highest risk factors for ill-health in the EU. In the past, LSD has been used successfully to treat alcoholism, at a range of dosages, although alcoholics who experienced a transcendent state during their session were far more likely to demonstrate a long term improvement in their conditions, and such states were induced more commonly with higher doses. A review of old studies conducted in the 1960s and 1970s found that 59% of people reported lower levels of alcohol misuse following treatment, compared to 38% who received the placebo, which is as good as any current alcoholism treatments. Patients who experienced a profound sense of cosmic unity or ego death seemed to change their outlook on their addictions.

Alcoholics Anonymous co-founder Bill Wilson claimed his experience with LSD played an integral part in his recovery from alcoholism, and encouraged him to found AA. He didn't view LSD as a magic bullet for alcoholism, more of an ally that could set up a goal and incentive for recovery. A study published this year looking at many thousands of people found no association between psychedelics and mental health issues. In fact there were less mental health issues in the psychedelic using group, and lifetime LSD use was correlated with less psychiatric hospital visits and a lower use of prescription drugs.

Recent studies have used psilocybin in the treatment of alcoholism and tobacco addiction. These are ongoing pilot studies with a small sample size so far but the results are encouraging and further research is certainly warranted. Of the four people who have been treated for tobacco addiction with psilocybin, one year after treatment three were no longer smoking and one had gone from a pack a day to one cigarette a week. Despite the small number of people in this study so far, this is encouraging, as the average success rate of quitting smoking is between 20 - 40%.

Psychedelics act in a number of different ways in the brain that impact addiction. They act on the receptors in the brain associated with drug seeking behaviour, while reducing blood flow to areas of the brain associated with emotional processing and higher function that tend to be overactive in depressives. This perhaps put the brakes on the negative circular thought patterns associated with addiction. The temporary chaotic state induced by psychedelics seems to weaken reinforced brain connections and dynamics and the experience provides a window of reflection where people can view their life and addiction issues from a wider perspective. People who were more successful in quitting smoking had higher 'mystical experience' scores, and in other studies, the psilocybin induced mystical experience was found to cause positive changes in measures of life satisfaction and well being, as well as long term personality change, particularly in openness. This compromises personality traits such as placing value in aesthetics, emotion, openness to new experiences and a curiosity to further knowledge. It seems that this experience and the change in values and outlook also plays a key role in the anti-addiction effects of psychedelics such as psilocybin.

An increasing number of therapists are using ayahuasca in the treatment of substance addiction, and there is a growing research interest in this area. There are numerous positive subjective reports from people who have self medicated with ayahuasca to treat addiction, and participants in studies have reported positive lasting psychological and behavioural changes. Addiction expert Dr Gabor Maté views ayahuasca working on addiction in multiple ways; by allowing users to see the baggage associated with their addiction and appreciate it does not have to be a part of them, and by allowing them a positive experience of love for the self. Recent neuroimaging research on ayahuasca have found evidence of changes in brain structure in long term users, associated with positive changes in behaviour and feelings of life satisfaction, so changes in neuroplasticity within the brain may play a role in its anti-addictive effect. Ayahuasca also causes a serotonin up regulation that may have anti-depressant qualities, assisting with enacting life change post session.

Moreover, past studies looking at members of the União de Vegetal (UDV) Church revealed they felt ayahuasca had a profound impact on their lives. Many reported they were better able to see destructive behaviour patterns, and there was a tendency to discontinue alcohol, tobacco, cocaine and other drug addictions. It is also interesting to note that an appreciable proportion of long term ayahuasca users had suffered from alcoholism and depression prior to joining the UDV. In British Colombia ayahuasca has been used with success in addiction treatment among indigenous people there by Dr Gabor Maté, and in Peru it has been used to successfully treat cocaine addiction, notably in a therapeutic community setting at the Takiwasi Center, with future addiction research planned there.

Cannabis may play a role in the treatment of addictions. Both THC and cannabidiol (CBD) have been found to act as neuroprotective antioxidants against the effects of excessive alcohol use and neuro-degeneration of the white matter of the brain. Cannabis has been suggested as a much safer substitution treatment for alcoholism, cocaine and opiate addiction. Recent research has found CBD to markedly reduce cigarette consumption in smokers, and it may reduce cravings with other substances.

Unfortunately, at present, all classical psychedelics are considered Class A or Schedule 1 substances, deemed to have a high potential for abuse and no accepted medical use. However various psychedelic agents have been used by different cultures in different parts of the world to successfully treat addiction and other afflictions, and there is an ever expanding body of evidence to suggest their efficacy in this area. Draconian laws and numerous regulatory and financial hurdles currently stand in the way of any researchers hoping to work with these substances. This could be preventing the treatment of a condition that exerts a vast cost on many human lives, and on society as a whole.

CHAPTER 12

The LSD Trial

by Toby Slater

After passing the screening I was offered the opportunity to take part in the trial, which would involve two visits to Cardiff separated by a period of two weeks. One visit would be placebo, the other LSD. The study would involve brain-scanning and brain-imaging using the very latest fMRI and MEG technology to ascertain what is actually happening in the brain under the influence of LSD.

When administered intravenously the effects of LSD are much quicker than via oral ingestion - anytime between 5 and 15 minutes. Almost at once I began to feel odd: from nervous flutters to various tingling sensations. My sense of balance and perspective was almost immediately affected. The preparatory scanner noises were strange but I felt relaxed and by the time I was brought out of the tube my visual perspectives were becoming increasingly bizarre, as if I'd shrunk or simultaneously grown in size - a perceptual contradiction which made the simple act of sitting up quite problematic. The floor felt soft and rubbery and so too the chair which I made my way to.

Once I sat down things felt more manageable despite the fact that the LSD experience had begun to intensify. It became apparent to me that the normal way we experience the world is entirely dependent on clearly regimented neuro-scientific factors. If these factors are altered, the world-view that we normally experience becomes fragile and in flux. All around me the dimensions of the room seemed crooked. Right angles and parallel lines didn't appear to meet at the places where they normally should, rather like an Escher painting. The contours of the room appeared to move and stretch and hard surfaces seemed soft and malleable.

I felt a tremendous euphoria slowly rising in me, accompanied by a general amusement at the world at large – the world one normally takes for granted. The seriousness of the austere environment at once seemed pompous, absurd and cartoonish. Ordinary reality and its normally sealed surfaces, codes and conventions seemed to break open and become increasingly plastic. Even the very grains of the walls seemed to vibrate as if I could see into the fundamentals of its atomic structure.

During this period I was sat with Dr Robin Carhart-Harris, the trial co-ordinator; and Dr Tim Williams, a colleague and psychiatrist. They both became very amusing to me - caricatures of their previous forms. We also had some interesting dialogue but the problem was I had too many thoughts and found it hard to not veer off on conversational tangents. My mind seemed expanded, buzzing with 'aliveness' yet also in a state of entropy, in the sense that I felt I could see and think about anything, so therefore concentrating on any one thing in a systematic linear fashion was a challenge.

Around this time physical transformations became even more apparent. The room took on the appearance of an oil painting that was still wet, and the two co-ordinators began to physically morph and change in various ways. Tim seemed to change into various famous people, and at the same time seemed archetypal and increasingly strange. Robin, whom I was more familiar with, greatly amused me and his face appeared to be constantly melting. I recall one particular moment when he rummaged in the pockets of his combat shorts, which seemed unfathomably deep as if they might contain the entire content of the universe.

Robin asked me to sign some papers. Such a regular action, which we do so often, seemed bizarre like a silly game. I viewed this activity like an alien might or an individual from a remote tribe who wasn't familiar with such customs. The physical act of signing my name was also difficult: the pen felt rubbery and bendy, the table uneven and the paper's surface felt like water. The ink glided across the paper as smooth as velvet and I remember finding it funny that the pen 'knew what to say'.

Robin explained how to answer the scaling exercises which I would be presented with inside the scanner. On placebo two weeks ago the questions seemed logical and reasonable, yet on LSD they seemed absurd and ridiculous, as if somehow trying to measure and quantify an unfathomably abstract experience with crude objects like a ruler and calculator. I felt in that instant that this is what is so limiting about our mechanistically-orientated rationalist culture.

Mendel Kaelen, a Dutch PhD student working on the study, came into the room to fit the light beads to my face, which are necessary apparatus for the scanning process. His 'Dutchness' was strikingly apparent, so too the interaction between him and Robin, who by contrast seemed quintessentially English. This led to a conversation about cultural stereo-types and I began to reflect on how cultural conditioning is rather like a computer software programme: all of us have our cultural programme uploaded by the various environments and 'main-frame' systems we are raised in.

The overall experience was like having stepped out the limiting enclo-sure of ordinary consciousness into an unveiled new reality. The LSD experience is rather like entering the backstage area of a theatre - the per-formance taking place on the stage being 'normal reality'. The psychedelic state is like the backstage area because one feels one is able to experience how the presentation of ordinary reality is organised and directed. I felt like I could see behind the mechanisms we usually take for granted. I had the sensation that the normal and necessary filters had been removed. This felt liberating and, combined with the physical sensations I was experiencing, created euphoric feelings of near ecstasy. These sensations were further-more accompanied by increasingly bizarre visual changes from melting Dali-like surfaces to brilliant cascading geometric patterns in the carpets and the walls. Everything around me seemed to breathe and pulsate, lit up with a fantastic gleam - a light source that bounded off any surface I focused on.

If I closed my eyes I could see brilliant phosphorescence: a source of energy that burst into any manifestation I cared to consider. I can remem-ber thinking that I was not ready for this inner world yet so opened my eyes again to the gleaming outer world transforming before me. I recall reflect-ing on the immense power of these chemicals which can catalyse so much material that exists within all of us at any one time but is normally inacces-sible. I also contemplated why an alkaloid might exist in nature, the psilo-cybin mushroom, which is similar in chemical structure to LSD. It fits into the neurotransmitter perfectly like a chemical key; making manifest a new perception of reality. Why do these chemicals exist in nature if not to reveal something, or be used for a higher purpose?

My mind seemed incredibly agile, able to fly from one subject to another outside normal linear and often pedestrian constraints. My brain felt like a nerve-centre connected to the entire universe; with this came the notion that we are all one consciousness simply experiencing itself subjec-tively. This idea seemed a likely possibility in the state of mind I was in. It was as if I'd gone into a room, a mansion with endless windows looking out onto multiple vistas. The mansion was the breadth of the human mind itself and the combination of possible experiences. I felt like I could peer out through any window into different realities. I was no longer a prisoner of my own limited point-of-view i.e. the view from the single window of the self.

It was time to go through to the scanner room, just before however I went to the toilet. This simple ordinary activity was not an easy experience. The environment of the bathroom was a like a world in itself. It seemed super brightly lit and clinical with all kinds of unfamiliar switches, cords and buttons. I also lost all track of time and felt like I was in there for an eternity. My face in the mirror became a subtle shifting montage of various family portraits. I saw my father, mother, siblings, grandfather and children all within my own face. In retrospect this isn't as absurd as it sounds if we consider family genes, but it was a bizarre thing to actually 'see'.

Outside the bathroom cubicle the corridor carpets were swirling and squirming like a cross between frogspawn and the liquid shapes you see when you stare up at the sky in the summertime - probably liquid on the eyeball reinterpreted and fused over normal physical surfaces. I met Tim who handed me my bottle of mineral water, which suddenly felt very precious to me.

In the scan room I felt like I'd left the warm security of the previous phase. There was a definite shift in tone and mood. The environment now felt cold, clinical and deadly serious after the liberated euphoria of before. The scan operator, although pleasant, seemed remote and robotic compared to the friendly co-ordinators. The room itself was cold and had an air of menace about it - at least that's how I perceived it. There was a strange rhythmic breathing noise in the background, which sounded ominous and foreboding. It retrospect it must have been the energy source of the scanner but that rational possibility was unobtainable for me at that moment.

I lay down onto the gurney and they fitted the headphones, heart monitor and the various straps and appendages. I remember looking up at Robin and Tim leaning over me and it felt like an archetypal death-bed scene. I said to Robin "This feels like the end of my life". Robin reassured me that this wasn't the case and that I would be absolutely fine. I tried to relax as I was fed slowly into the scanner tube.

The advised mantra was 'If in doubt float downstream' which reinforces the importance of letting go when faced with difficulty or uncertainty. With this in mind I was able to contain my anxiety. Deep inside the narrow confines the scan operator asked me if I was ok, his voice sounding from inside my headphones. I said I was ok and tried to relax by focusing on my breath and reassuring myself that I was in safe hands taking part in a rare and invaluable experience.

From behind my veil of calm I focused on how lucky I was, and how my normal 'ordinary life', to which I would soon return, was just fine. This however led me to wonder why on earth I would therefore want to experience this madness. I reflected how in my life I have often craved alien experiences outside of the norm, yet once there I can feel a momentary urge to return to safe confines. A good example is the feeling of culture shock in strange exotic places. I reassured myself that like the travelling experience, the strange and exotic would soon become manageable and enriching.

I was able to let go and drift inwards which was accompanied by an intense sensation of moving deeper into internal realms. Very soon I felt as if I'd travelled on a deep journey inwards beyond the normal parameters of time and space, like journeying into the depths of an internal cosmos.

I saw vast landscapes and panoramic vistas open up. I had the sensation I was flying blissfully over craggy mountain ranges rich with vegetation. This was accompanied by a weightless feeling of being free from the burdens and shackles of ordinary existence. I had the clear illuminating sense that I was beginning to see my life in all of its stages, colours and tones. I experienced an acute over-view: the sense that I understood and accepted so much that in normal consciousness is often hard to grasp and fathom. It felt like an insight into the higher order of things, even the organic laws of chaos. It was as if the filters or blinkers had been lifted off completely. The following expression came to me with a ring of clarity: 'the natural perfection of imperfection'.

After this intense feeling of unveiled existential freedom and acceptance - it is hard to recall how long it lasted - I felt a tangible remembrance of the safe confines of the life that I was leaving behind. Looking back now this backward glance was a definitive moment of the conflict that followed. It was also a pivotal moment which I could have been handled differently in a purely therapeutic environment. I did what I could however by telling myself to let go again. For a while I was able to do so successfully. I was still flying over landscapes but this time the topography of the territory had changed. It was now barren like a desert or the surface of the moon. The terrain now seemed to contain my entire life-story. All of my history, in terms of actual events, was buried beneath the surface.

A new shift occurred around this time; whilst before I'd felt like the 'first-person narrator' looking down upon the landscape like a kite, I began to feel like I had broken out of the confines of that ordinary viewpoint. I remember reassuring myself with a line from a William Blake poem where he describes the 'mind-forged manacles[1]' of how one normally sees and perceives; so too the famous quote about the doors of perception, which I shall quote in full especially because of the lesser known following line:

If the doors of perception were cleansed everything would appear to man as it is, infinite. For man has closed himself up, till he sees all things thro' narrow chinks of his cavern[2].

This experience therefore could be the ultimate liberation: the opening up of the 'narrow chinks' but the challenge was that it distinctively felt as if the kite's mooring - to the safe ground of my ordinary life - was becoming increasingly fragile. I knew from the literature that this is known as 'ego-dissolution'. I told myself I understood this, but my conceptual understanding is from an ego-bound notion of reality. From the psychedelic perspective, where subject and object was blurring, it became increasing hard to understand what was happening - my sense of self, the "I" that cognitively knows that it understands was itself dissolving.

Ego-dissolution and the fear of letting go was the crux of the difficulties that followed in the claustrophobic confines of the fMRI scanner. A conceptual understanding of the importance of letting go is a valuable life lesson, but a tangible realisation of the consequences of not letting go is a profound cautionary tale that I will never forget.

Yet the experience was primarily pleasurable: deeply sensory, existential and other-worldly. I felt like I was beach-combing a lunar landscape which had a luminous phosphorescent quality to it. The beach-combing became an archaeological dig at the site of my entire life story - I could fly in and out of various aspects and memories as if they were pods within the terrain.

I noticed the 'distraction' of the scanner noises - maybe they changed or simply my perception altered - which reminded me of my tethering to ordinary reality. The noises felt invasive and created visual bolts of lightning inside me occurring in time with the sound. I was then 'interrupted' by a voice in my ear asking if I was ok - the voice of the scan operator - collectively these aspects didn't help the process of letting go.

The voice of the scan operator caused me to open my eyes and I was shocked to realise the close confines of the environment again. It was as if I had completely forgotten about the reality of the scanner - the 'inner world' of my subconscious had over-ridden the external environment. I was asked by the computer to scale my experience.

I remember the scoring grids seemed totally inadequate in being able to capture the 'secret realities' I was experiencing, but I scored highly in the sense that my experience was off the scale. I remember it was difficult to operate the simple buttons as if it wasn't my body that I was operating. I told the operator I needed to come out for a time.

Coming out of the tube was like being reborn into another layer of the external world: a shocking shift of perspective from enclosed space to mass exposure. The co-ordinators asked me if I was ok. I said I was but that I wanted to come out now - coming out of the confines had made me realise how intense it was being inside. Quite understandably they needed to continue with the collection of data and so after being reassured I was guided back inside with the various attachments in place.

The screen above my head told me to shut my eyes again and I distinctly remember being frightened at the prospect of re-entering the inner world again. Whilst it had been incredible and other-worldly it was also existentially frightening. I can remember wanting a guide to help me navigate my way through this complex terrain. I felt very alone and didn't want to go back inside ('out there') again. This feeling was also accompanied by the sense that I just didn't want to let go anymore. I wanted instead to return to the safe shores of the ordinary mind. I then feared, and not for the last time, that perhaps I would never return to those shores: a disturbing potential aspect of the psychedelic experience.

I remember disturbing images coming to me: brutal images of war, others grotesquely sexual and pornographic, mixed with montages of imprisonment. The images burst before my eyes like flash-bulbs going off. On reflection some of this may have been fuelled by topical media threads of the time: the Syrian crisis; the endless sexual abuse scandals, and the recent imprisonment of foreign journalists in Egypt. Perhaps these images also became entangled within my own feelings of 'imprisonment' within the scanner. I came out of the scanner briefly again to try and air my concerns. The co-ordinators reassured me and I went back in.

This time music was played. The track was soothing and turned the experience into a clichéd '60's psychedelic moment by which I mean the vibe of the song reminded me of The Beatles 'Tomorrow Never Knows'. It wasn't so much the essence of the music itself, as it was quite different, but it created that concept in me. The Beatles song is of course about LSD. The music also reminded me of chill-out Café Del Mar soundtracks from the late '90s. I was able to move inside the sinews of the song itself, which was a welcome distraction from the invasive alien sounds of the scanner. That said I could still hear them blasting through me, which felt like an electric drill, each blast again accompanied by a lightning bolt.

The situation became increasingly challenging with difficult life and family issues emerging in greater clarity. Some of the issues were informed by new events in the few days before I returned to Cardiff. I had wondered if these issues might have been a problem but I took the decision that I would be able to deal with them.

I began to experience a particular private memory, which was something I thought I had previously processed. Yet inside the scanner, having my brain 'photographed', it felt like everyone in the world knew about it which created an intensely paranoid feeling. I wanted to discuss it but couldn't due to its complexity; due to the fact that the co-ordinators didn't know me, and of course the obvious isolation. The tension built and built as all of the memories of my life then seemed to cascade towards me.

LSD, as much as it is understood, is a catalysing agent which acts as an amplifier of material that is present in the unconscious mind. This certainly rings true as my account testifies but also because I had a vivid and tangible recollection of a reoccurring childhood nightmare.

The scenario of the nightmare: I would find myself standing on the brink of a great precipice looking out across a giant chessboard. As a child I would look out at this endless board knowing that I had to make a move which would have eternal and everlasting consequences. I had never been able to understand or interpret the dream yet I've never forgotten the cataclysmic sense of impending terror that the dream would create. I hadn't experienced the nightmare since I was a child but under the influence of LSD that very landscape opened up within me - a terrifying experience which is hard to express. The experience of psychedelics making the unconscious mind manifest is further supported by the following quote concerning mescaline:

> *The most compelling insight of that day was that this awesome recall had been brought about by a fraction of a gram of a white solid, but that in no way whatsoever could it be argued that these memories had been contained within the white solid. Everything I had recognized came from the depths of my memory and my psyche. I understood that our entire universe is contained in the mind and the spirit. We may choose not to find access to it, we may even deny its existence, but it is indeed there inside us, and there are chemicals that can catalyse its availability[3].*

The early onset of 'ego dissolution' became more and more pronounced. The metaphorical kite string, which tethered me to the ground of my identity, seemed to no longer be there. From previous studies with psilocybin, neuroscientists believe that the experience of 'ego dissolution' relates to a decrease of blood flow in the region of the brain known as the Default Mode Network - a fundamental connector hub or hierarchal organising principle better known as the 'ego'. In the psychedelic state this region appears to go 'offline'. It is analogous to a capital city shutting down, or a conductor walking off stage leaving the orchestra to play on without guidance, order or direction. The tide of information without the normal filters of the DMN can then be experienced as 'too much reality' without a discerning (ego) agent to organise or make sense of it[4].

Ego-dissolution can be perceived as a blissful archetypal 'spiritual' experience or, if coupled with anxiety and unpleasant circumstances, the very opposite. Aldous Huxley in *The Doors of Perception* (1954) described the Default Mode Network as a 'reducing valve', an idea he borrowed from Henri Bergson, and which has an evolutionary basis[5].

Our minds have evolved to filter out information for practical survival purposes. A pure survivalist mode perhaps supersedes contemplating beauty by looking at the world in slow meditation when there are crops to tend to and mouths to feed. At the same time Huxley and others argued that mankind is potentially in a state of crisis from having filtered out too much. It is as if we have lost something vital in a very critical sense: we've become too rational, blinded by the motors of technological advancement, economic growth and consumption.

To live fully to our potential perhaps we need to cleanse our perception with a renewed sense of wonder and reverence. I believe that we need beauty as nourishment for the soul, which is the consolation prize to counter all the ugliness, pain and suffering in the world. This is not a plea to returning to the pure irrationality of magical thinking but perhaps regaining the essential delight in the beauty and mystery of simple things. Huxley calls this the 'Mind At Large' - perhaps catalysed by a reduction of blood to the DMN which formally in classical times was the preserve of seers, mystics, and visionaries of the ages. Albert Hofmann hoped his 'elixir' could renew our wonder of the world and rescue civilisation from the dour trajectory pure materialism appears to be leading us towards[6].

My experience of ego-dissolution was categorised by extremes: an initial and lasting existential phase of flying in and out of various life events and being able to see them with apocalyptic clarity. As described this 'unveiling' was at first blissful and a tremendous release, but soon after I felt a sudden and urgent need to return to the here and now. It was then that I realised that I had no clear means to guide me back and furthermore no sense of a conceptual "I" to return to.

The next phase of my experience was characterised by an increased state of confusion. As described I had been previously able to look down upon various life phases; flying in and out of the 'pods'. Yet now they seemed to dissolve, and I could no longer separate myself from them as an observer. The divide between subject and object seemed to completely disappear. The sensation was like merging into a borderless mass of space; an infinite and free-flowing source of energy without divides, organising principles, or means of categorisation. It was completely overwhelming: a feeling of being lost and adrift in the endless chaos of time. Without a clearly defined sense of identity – an "I" to observe and experience - time itself becomes an endless and unfathomable entity. Perhaps this is its true nature when one is freed from the ego-mind?

The findings from the recent psilocybin trials support the fact that I was experiencing entropic confusion[7]. In mechanistic terms the useful 'fixed' circuits or systems of my brain had become temporarily fluid and plastic. My grasp of memory, time and the perception of various life events were in a state of flux. My 'objective' view was reduced to a molten mass of reflections, a diaspora of events in what felt like an eternity.

Attempting to cling on is a key aspect: the 'trip switch' was my sense of doubt. Whilst I could talk myself around at first as the LSD experience intensified I couldn't let go in the scanner with all that had come to the surface. It was this very aspect of clinging on that catalysed the conflicting angst. Holding on during 'ego-dissolution' feels like dying and is therefore the ultimate existential crisis. It almost redefines that term as the ultimate high-wire psychological moment. I believe if I'd had a guide in a therapeutic context outside of the scanner the result might have been very different however.

Czech Psychiatrist Stanislav Grof, who conducted extensive LSD research over many years prior to prohibition, found the imagery of death and rebirth central to a certain stage of the LSD experience. I don't believe I reached completion of the 'death' stage, nor did I get to experience the full catharsis of rebirth but I did glimpse significant aspects of these stages as the following quote supports:

> *The subject finds him or herself awash in the contents of the personal unconscious, confronting everything from sexual and religious taboos to childhood fears and family relationships. Often this involves consciously re-experiencing one's own birth trauma (even details unknown to the subject) followed by catharsis – a release or breakthrough into transpersonal realms*[8].

I knew I had to get out of the scanner once and for all, which was followed by a powerful urge to leave the clinical trial environment altogether and get home to my family. The urge felt primal and it is hard to do justice to how I felt in that moment. Perhaps I was experiencing aspects of the 'birth trauma' that Grof describes. Either way I believed I had gone too far and I had to abandon the trial and be 'reborn' to save my own skin and be there for my family. The underlying fear was that I would never return from these wild shores, which was amped up by the fact that I couldn't be sure what 'time line' I was now living in.

The 'aloneness' of the scanner became unbearable. I felt that I was in serious jeopardy if I was to continue. It was like a sci-fi nightmare scenario - think *Twelve Monkeys* or *The Matrix*, a feeling of pure undulated terror. A feeling that no-one around me understood my deep existential emergency.

I pressed the squeeze-ball again. The scan operator's voice asked if I was alright. I said I needed to come out. I felt terribly exposed again, lying on the slab after the enclosure of the scanner with concerned or 'irritated' faces looking at me. It felt like being born in a very visceral way. I also felt like an overexposed film emerging from a camera, which was very unpleasant. I began to physically remove some of the various electrodes and wires as I felt my entire being was in jeopardy.

Sitting up I noticed something significant which came to be critical: an apparent difference of opinion between the two co-ordinators in how to respond to my situation.

Robin was on one side of the gurney looking frustrated - in retrospect a totally understandable reaction for the trial organiser needing to collect data, which I was essentially forfeiting. Tim, the psychiatrist, stood on the other side and seemed to recognise my urgent need to get out of the environment and the situation. The physical separation of the two figures emphasised their difference of opinion. Robin noticed this and moved to the same side as Tim - an astute move. At the same time I saw this move too.

From then on two insights occurred: I felt I was a mere 'lab rat', and the difference of opinion with Robins' attempt to correct it (or in my mind conceal it) ended the prior trust or bond. This was a significant shift and one which characterised what was to follow.

The co-ordinators helped me off the slab and let me leave the scanning room. I remember asking if I would ever get back to normality. They reassured me that I would. I wanted to believe them but 'normality' was an unobtainable and unfathomable concept to consider so my question and their answer was beyond comprehension.

I was handed my bottle of water and led back to the mock scan room where it had all begun. This was a wise tactic as it was where I'd felt safe. What was frightening was the room now seemed different and alien. The mock-scanner was huge and bone-like; a giant fossil. It also appeared to breathe. I turned away and began to feel totally out of reach from this point on - perhaps as a consequence of having lost 'trust' in the coordinators. They appeared to watch me 'suspiciously' when in retrospect it was simply the concern of trying to reach me and contain an unpredictable situation. I felt like I had gone insane, and I certainly felt like I was acting so.

The co-ordinators physical appearances transformed again correlating with my altered beliefs about them. Their faces mutated into shimmers of florid pigmentation. Robin appeared 'wolf-like' which greatly frightened me. I decided not to focus on them and turned inwards seeking some kind of refuge.

For a time I was lost to the inner world of my own mind: a complex matrix of narratives past, present and future. I was desperately trying to figure out where I was *i.e.* my place in time, and how I would get out and get back. It was like an impenetrable puzzle that I had to solve. I remember the experience was like being stuck in a maddening loop.

At the same time I was disturbed by the difficult family issues which I felt I couldn't talk to the co-ordinators about - as they knew nothing about them as I hadn't chosen to share it. I was unable or unwilling to explain them. This whole phase was characterised by a feeling of unbearable conflict and being unable to 'break the spell' to transcend the complex difficulty I was in.

The co-coordinators both attempted to engage with me, asking if I was ok and whether I wanted to talk about what I was experiencing. I said I was ok to placate them but in truth I was in a catastrophic emergency: I didn't know where I was, how I'd got here, or even why I was dressed in medical scrubs with a cannula fixed. The environment and the medical paraphernalia increased the idea that perhaps my notions of home and getting back were illusions and that in fact I was a mental hospital in-mate.

I attempted to test my theory by saying that I needed to go home which was met quite naturally with a 'not right now' response. This increased the paranoid fear that I was in fact mad. I remember sitting still with a dry throat, trying to drink water from a bottle that seemed like it was made of water itself. I was bereft yet continued to try to untangle the existential twist that I was in.

On reflection this episode gives me a deep heart-felt empathy for anyone who has experienced a psychotic episode, or suffers the bewildering confusions of paranoid schizophrenia. I can also empathise with the Alzheimer's sufferer or the elderly person who wants to 'go home' but is told they can't by care-home staff.

Robin played some calming music on his phone: a cinematic soundtrack with piano and strings as I recall. Normally I respond positively to music but in this instance it didn't connect. The well-intentioned act of being played music felt contrived; an artificial reason to keep me in this bizarre situation. I had the terrible burdened feeling of waiting for something to happen, for something to shift or change - but I didn't know what it was that I was waiting for. I then asked to change out of the scrubs that I was wearing.

Upstairs I was shown my clothes. It felt strange to see these familiar items: like a costume that I wear to play the character that is me. On many levels this observation is accurate because the style and presentation one chooses - one's aesthetic identity - is entirely constructed. I struggled to get the clothes over my cannula which I was told I couldn't remove yet, which made me think that they intended to give me more LSD.

I recall getting my phone out: this ever-present piece of technology which, like most people, is where I store a lot of personal information and is my link to the outside world. It looked totally alien like an obsolete relic from another era. This reinforces the notion that the psychedelic experience deconditions the mind; the familiar becomes unfamiliar. This is an incredibly important experience: to see the world anew, free from preconditioned symbols, signs and signifiers. This moment is the access point or window that could be utilised by a therapist. It is the portal into aspects of self that are stuck, rigid or in need of unravelling. The deconditioned mind allows the chance to begin again; to reboot, reconfigure and change ingrained habits or behaviours.

I accepted some food and asked if I could eat it near some daylight. On the way to a seated area I watched the receptionists performing their clerical office procedures under artificial light, which appeared robotic and devoid of meaning. Once sat down I wondered if I was in Hammersmith - where I'd done the screening for the trial. But upon looking out at the strange world beyond the glass I saw a sign for Cardiff University. It made no sense to me that I was in Cardiff, a city which has some personal significance to me, which furthered my confused 'lost in time' predicament.

Trying to eat a sandwich was difficult because I could barely swallow the food as a result of anxiety. Robin's appearance also became increasingly sinister. His features becoming 'wolf like' once again. Deconstructing this now it must have been a combination of his beard and my interpretation of his facial expressions: furrowed uncertainty about how to proceed with unpredictability, which I read as suspicion and danger. He represented a Jungian archetype of threat. This led to me to consider 'Steppenwolf' by Hermann Hesse - which may have been a semantic link because of the 'wolf 'of the title - but perhaps there was a deeper lateral connection because the novel was a bible for the 1960s psychedelic counter-culture and deals with themes of madness and rationality, and the conscious and unconscious mind.

After considering my predicament and seeing no possible end to the confusion I decided I needed to take practical measures. I had to leave and so abruptly swung my bag onto my shoulder and made a swift exit out of the building. I recall being hit by a barrage of sensory information: dazzling sunlight, bright colours, translucent blue sky and the unravelling chaos of a busy city street.

I heard Robin shout "Tim!" and almost instantly both co-ordinators appeared at either side of me. Tim said "As a doctor I cannot let you leave," which reinforced the sense that I was an escaping inmate from a mental institution. What is interesting is the cultural power a doctor possesses - my instant reaction which was to surrender to his demand despite being desperate to escape. I was led back in and down the stairs, which were like an Escher stair-case: a symbolic representation of the endless state I was in. I feared I was destined to repeat the same experience again: more LSD and more scanning for eternity.

Tim suggested fitting a cannula to my other arm which horrified me as surely this meant more LSD. He reassured me that it was the best means of supplying me with an anti-anxiety drug which would reduce the angst I was feeling. I agreed after some persuading and was administered a shot of Midazolam (a benzodiazepine). I don't recall what happened after as it knocked me out for about ten minutes.

When I came around I felt an immediate and over-whelming sense of relief: a return to the clear ego-bound constraints of organised reality. My mind state was still altered but the shifting sands of existential anxiety had stopped. It was essentially a rebirth following the mythic fragmentation of ego-dissolution.

A debrief followed allowing me to talk about what had happened, some of which was recorded for research purposes. I was able to make complete sense of the confusion I'd felt and had some fascinating discussions about some of the insights, including the chessboard nightmare I used to have as a child. I also talked about an aspect of childhood and my religious upbringing, concepts such as the divided self by the psychologist R.D Laing, and the work of mythologist Joseph Campbell.

My psychedelic experience certainly makes sense in the context of the mythic structure of the 'Hero's Journey'. This isn't a new revelation; the sixties saw Campbell's classic work of the heroes' quest reinterpreted by LSD users. Put simply the story or "monomyth" which all human beings in all cultures embark upon is the quest to discover the essence of who we really are[9]. In psychoanalytical terms this involves the narrative of facing oneself in all its guises, especially the inherent conflicts of the unconscious, and returning with new insights is the underlying story of all our lives, and certainly an insight I glimpsed on LSD. The psychedelic experience mirrors the hero's quest - a departure from the world of everyday experience, followed by a crisis of initiation (death/rebirth), and eventual return[10].

One could argue that I failed the initiation, or it was 'interrupted' or annulled by the anti-anxiety injection. The extreme psychedelic effects certainly ended prematurely. I believe my decision to leave the fMRI environment was the correct one however. I may also have fared much better if I had been able to communicate my fears and concerns. Most significant however is the broad understanding that I was left with - the 'boon' or treasure of insight that I took away with me in the aftermath.

During the debrief I recall Robin saying that he'd identified a sense of conflict in me from when we had first met and that perhaps some of these aspects were amplified during the session. I accept that observation as there are conflicts within me that are worthy of greater reflection. Perhaps we all contain aspects of struggle and tension and that it is our life's journey to resolve, accept or transcend them. The starting point is surely an awareness of the source. Psychedelics provide a direct confrontation with the source as my experience testifies – which supports the notion that a therapeutic environment with skilled guides could prove to be transformational.

The Trial

An awareness of doors opening in the walls, nodes cascading out;
Sweet laughter seeps as words break from their shells.
Colours humming their melodies under deep pulses of light,
The right angles of the room wronged as faces melt and morph,
We talk about the sound of cities and the imprints they left on us.
Until surfaces soften and breathe following the trail of grains,
Hushed like falling petals into deepening liquid floors.
The Shangri-La disintegrates as I'm led to my resting place.
Strapped to the slab and plugged-in: mummified meat for the machine.
With blanket and headphones, and a fist full of squeeze-ball,
I'm fed into the scanner staring upwards to white letters,
The words on the black screen demand I close my eyes.
Confines of space open up as I follow a shimmering inroad,
Rushing through the underground, smiling as if I know the secret,
My face a thousand pictures, connections lighting the dark,
Psychic photos mapping flashing fission of mind,
The first-person narrator goes off line as vistas open wide:
Plains of fibrous light with every flaw and gulley revealed,
Flying over the order of chaos - the perfection of imperfection.
Divinity in the kites-eye view until the line grows tight,
Fear of tethers fraying as a thousand narratives unwind,
Below a mosaic of bones in endless cemeteries of silence.
I went out so far within - to the inside where we all begin,
But I couldn't hold the secrets; the weight was too much,
I worried for the cost - I had to get out, I had to get back.
Only I was lost, plugged into the veins of the cosmos.
A thousand different lives, a thousand different times.
I knew I was lucky, that I was in love, but then "I" dissolved.
The walled-in part vanished as time lines burst to speech bubbles.
"I love you", "Where are you"? But where was I? Lost in the wires,

With the hiss of a thousand snakes, jungle rattles and broken breath.
Reaching for the surface where there was only depth,

Urging for dry land in the eternal melt: chaos of time unveiled,
Coloured sand filled endless vials like grains of television screen.
A thousand windows reflecting too much sky: a grand whole of shame.
No horizons lines to frame or offer breaks and stops,
Only the fizz of wires and the ghosts of faces in catacombs.
Too many stones to turn on a chessboard of infinite moves,
The eternal consequence of choice: same old puzzle, same old pieces -
For a moment it all came together until jeopardy dawned in bold.
A bid to escape the lab with my burdened bag of tricks,
With uniform and mask fixed the treasures at once lost to me;
I could not leave and was led back down vertigo steps,
To the mock rooms for further cycles of eternity,
Breaking speed to freeze-frame, smashed by slap of sleep;
Yet the glimpse of the infinity-machine still brims.

CHAPTER 13

Archaidelics

Amplifiers of the Archetypal

by Tim Read

The psyche in its deepest reaches participates in a form of existence beyond space and time and thus partakes of what is inadequately and symbolically described as eternity.

Carl Jung[1]

The Guru Effect

The night before Ram Dass met his guru for the first time, he was sitting outdoors in the starlit Indian night, thinking about his mother who had died the year before. The next day he had an unexpected encounter with a holy man, who seemed to know exactly what he had been thinking. This ragged old man told him that the previous night he had been under the stars, thinking about his mother. 'She died last year, she had a big stomach, she died of spleen'.

Somehow, this elderly Indian, living simply in the mountains, had a way of accessing accurate information about him that he could not have gained by any comprehensible means. He seemed to exist on a different level entirely, he had 'siddhis' – supernatural powers and he also radiated an extraordinary compassion. Ram Dass was shaken to his core by this realisation and describes a sense of relief, of 'coming home'. He knew that his search was over at last. Psychedelics had opened the doors of perception for him, but to his great frustration, the doors kept swinging shut again; he had learned that psychedelics could only take you so far. He knew that he had finally found someone for whom the doors were perpetually open.

Sometime later, the holy man wanted to try Ram Dass's 'special medicine', so on two separate occasions he took a high dose of LSD; 900 micrograms, and nothing happened to him. LSD apparently had no effect on him—whatsoever[2].

One of the many unusual qualities of psychedelics is the way in which the effect varies according to the dosage. In higher doses, there may be transpersonal experiences involving a transcendence of the ego with high-grade and potentially life-changing numinous experiences. In lower doses, as used in psycholytic psychotherapy, ego function is retained but modified in such a way that the fault lines of the psyche, the challenging personal issues and intra psychic conflicts, are brought into a brighter focus with amplification of meaning and intensity. In doses that are too small to exert a noticeable effect (microdosing), there may be a cognitive and creativity enhancing effect[3]. Any model that seeks to fully explain the effect of psychedelics needs to explain these qualities but also the phenomenon described by Ram Dass. Let us call it the guru effect.

Psychedelic - Archaidelic

The term psychedelic, meaning 'mind manifesting', has been used since the late 1950s but perhaps the term *archaidelic* is more appropriate if these drugs create their effect by manifesting a specifically *archetypal* layer of psyche. This is a significant distinction; psyche generally refers to the mind of an individual person while archetypes are *transpersonal* constructs extending beyond the individual psyche into a deeper layer of consciousness, perhaps even a cosmos that seems to be organized around meaning.

To explore this further, we need to clarify the nature of archetype, what it is and what it is not. I use the term archetype in the Jungian tradition to describe an underlying or deeper order involving a heightened intensity of meaning. This is different to the use of the term *stereotype*, which refers to a superficial rather than a deeper order and which does not amplify meaning. A stereotype has meaning but an archetype has Meaning. The concept of concentrated meaning is absolutely fundamental to an understanding of archetypes; thus an archetypal experience holds a meaning that invariably evokes a sense of awe. This sense of awe, which we may call a *numinous* experience, may be deeply positive and beautiful or deeply negative and dread filled.

Various quantum physicists have speculated about the role of consciousness and meaning in the physical universe – for Sir James Jeans; *'the universe begins to look more like a great thought than a great machine*[4]*'*. David Bohm, a protégé of Einstein, proposed a model of the universe where meaning is not separate from matter at all - but comes from the same fundamental stuff from which matter emerges. Bohm introduced the term *soma-significance* to highlight the unity between meaning (significance) and matter (soma) and proposed a deeper structure of universe, the *implicate order* where soma-significance could be infinitely concentrated to ever greater levels of complexity. Bohm considered that significance was unfolded from the implicate order to structure the everyday world in which we live.

Bohm's ideas are complicated, but introduce the crucial concept of meaning as a fifth dimension that can be experienced with various octaves of intensity[5]. Aldous Huxley gave us the notion of the brain as a 'reducing valve' to reduce the intensity of meaning to an acceptable range thus preventing us from being overwhelmed with information that is irrelevant to our everyday task. Huxley found that there was a much greater range of meaning that he termed 'mind at large', which our reducing valve filtered to a 'measly trickle[6]'. Huxley was powerfully influenced by his experiences with psychedelics, which remain the most accessible way of bypassing this valve.

If we consider a spectrum of meaning from the very low (as in inanimate objects) to the extraordinarily intense experiences of meaning that characterise the psychedelic experience, we can conceive of archetypes as the great weather systems of meaning under which we play out our little lives. According to this perspective, we are not simply biological machines existing in a mechanical universe, but much more complex organisms with roots tapping into the deeper mind stuff of the implicate order. Perhaps there is a participation between our brain and a transpersonal form of consciousness; a meeting between two forms of mind. Thus archetype mingles inextricably with our bio-psycho-social form and we live our lives on the cusp of that mingling.

There is no measurable scientific evidence confirming the central role of meaning in the physical universe, but we may find our own personal evidence in the form of *synchronicity*. A synchronicity is a meaningful coincidence; a correspondence between an inner experience and an event in the external world that has a profound meaning for the person who experiences it. A synchronicity is an ah-ha moment, it provokes a sense of awe, it is a numinous experience to a greater or lesser degree. It is an awakening to an awareness of a deeper order.

Archetypes come in flavours; older, polytheistic civilisations named them as their Gods. Classical Greece brought archetypes to life in a particularly personal and vivid manner showing how gods such as Zeus, Athena, Apollo, Aphrodite, Poseidon, Dionysus and many more exerted their influence over the world of men. Joseph Campbell, an expert on comparative mythology, suggested that myths act as a conduit for archetypal energies emanating from the cosmos, forming our spiritual heritage and shaping the great themes of humanity. Archetypes flow through our modern lives in similar cultural experiences with mythic qualities whether films, games, festivals or socio-political currents[7]. So if psychedelics amplify a specifically archetypal layer of psyche, it is inevitable that the archetypal oceans into which we dive will crystalize sometimes into mythic themes.

Archetypes are permanent and unchanging whereas anything that we can see, hear or touch in the physical world is transient. Physical forms degrade while archetypes do not degrade. An archetype is a universal principle, an essence, an idea that gives the visible world its form and meaning. Everything in our material world has an eternal unchanging form; courage, lust, evil, weather, a tree, a circle, even a chair. Diluted images of the archetypal form are made available to us through our sensory and cognitive apparatus. Something is beautiful precisely to the extent that it participates in the archetype of Beauty[8]. A beautiful person is informed by beauty but does not possess it. Physical beauty will fade but Beauty itself persists. Our idea of beauty is interpreted through the lens of our sensory system and cognitive apparatus but Beauty is independent of the physical domain. All the major themes of our human existence, the feelings, the yearnings, the totality of our emotional world could be understood in this way. The archetype is the unknowable form with a dimension that we cannot really comprehend, but we can see the archetypal images with varying degrees of intensity.

Archetypes flow though us; they are expressed through the hardware that is our body, our nervous system and our sense organs. If we are indeed influenced by an archetypal ocean with tides, currents, waves and undertows, then this may be more active – or *penetrant* - in some people than others and we may be more receptive to different archetypal flavors at different times.

The degree of *archetypal penetrance* is highly variable. Sometimes the intensity of archetypal penetrance is overwhelming for the psyche and the overdose of meaning causes a crisis. Some of us may have an innate or genetic predisposition for high archetypal penetrance (HAP) states – this may cause one of those archetypal crises that are classified as psychiatric conditions or it may predispose to a more creative or spiritual state. Some psychotropic drugs increase archetypal penetrance - with their use, the archetypal domain, is made more manifest so we can access the more concentrated and subtle forms of meaning that are usually denied to us.

The psychedelics/archaidelics that cause these high archetypal penetrance states have to be used skilfully of course, and we know that the principles of mindset, setting and integration are the fundamental determinants of outcome for any type of HAP state, archetypal crisis or psychedelic experience. Most people who take psychedelics these days are probably familiar with the principles of set and setting, but integration is often sub optimal. For those who want to move beyond recreational use towards therapeutic use or a serious growth path, a careful and thorough integration of the archetypal material is absolutely crucial.

Self and Shadow

The variety of archetypal experience is a huge topic, which I have tried to cover in *Walking Shadows*[9]. Here I will concentrate on the two elements of archetypal experience that I believe have most relevance for psychedelic experience – the *Self* and the *shadow*. The Jungian term Self can be confusing as it is entirely different to the personal self (or ego). The archetypal Self is at the apex of the pyramid of archetypes; indeed, it is beyond archetype, for it is the primal unity from which archetypes flow. The Self is comparable to the Hindu concept of Atman. For the Hindus, Atman pervades us utterly, as Krishna tells the hero of the Bhagavad Gita: 'I am the Self in the heart of every creature, Arjuna, and the beginning, middle and end of their existence[10]'. The Self never leaves us. It is our inner shining light.

The Self, like every archetype, is unknowable but we can taste the archetypal image of the Self in various ways. A high intensity image of the Self archetype may provide a peak experience, a memorable moment of cosmic union, but more commonly we may connect with Self with more modest experiences of illumination.

The shadow, on the other hand, is our dark side. It is the unseen reflection of the *persona*, which is the mask we use to present ourselves to the world. We all have a shadow; it is an inevitable part of being human; it is the part of our psyche that is around the corner and hidden from our sight. If light symbolises the visible aspect of consciousness, the shadow represents the part of ourselves that we do not choose to show to ourselves or anyone else. The shadow is not limited to unpleasant aspects of the repressed psyche, it may have great potential for creativity, for example, containing the repressed childlike playful side of the mature adult, or the feminine part of the masculine male and vice versa. It may even include the potential for love and altruism for people who have denied these aspects of their personalities. But generally, because it represents the qualities deemed unacceptable to us, the shadow is experienced as murky, lacking in morals, shameful and self-centred.

Monotheistic religions, from Zoroastrianism onwards, have been constructed around battles between archetypal good and evil, which could be understood as representing the tension between archetypal Self and archetypal shadow. If the Self stands for compassion, empathy and nurture, then the shadow stands for those parts of our individual and collective persona that has yet to be illuminated by those qualities. To make matters more complicated, the Self is at once light and dark, as much destructive as creative. So shadow is an integral part of Self and somehow destructive qualities need to be owned and integrated for the Self to be more fully realised. The encounter with and integration of the shadow is a crucial developmental step on our developmental journey. This may lead to a form of *ego death,* where redundant ego structures are shed with the emergence of a reborn ego permeated by Self. The resurrection myths of Baal, Osiris, Adonis, Dionysus and Christ point to this archetypal theme.

Archaidelics promise a potent encounter with these archetypal forces and the two classical features of the psychedelic experience are the spiritual experience and the bad trip. The experience of cosmic consciousness, or state of blissful unity, is, from the archetypal perspective, an encounter with Self, while the bad trip is an encounter with archetypal shadow.

At its most powerful, archetypal shadow can be extraordinarily difficult to bear and even harder to integrate. If we face our personal shadow, as we may choose do in psychotherapy, we confront, consider and integrate the aspects of ourselves that may cause us shame and distress. In a psychedelic experience these emotions will be amplified so that we experience them with archetypal intensity. These feelings may be extraordinarily powerful, with pervasive feelings of existential evil, destructiveness and despair. The archetypal wind fans the flame of our pain; we may even feel the pain of the entirety of humanity. These are the situations where we really need a sitter. What is less obvious is that it is often these bad trip scenarios where there is most potential for growth and development – but we have to work at it. Integration is crucial. People with a history of trauma or challenging emotional experiences will be more likely to revisit those emotional places in the high penetrance archetypal state of the psychedelic experience. Such states may be very complex and difficult to heal in everyday life or psychotherapy and it seems that, if well supported, HAP states may offer an opportunity to access and resolve some of the hidden areas in our psyche that can be so problematic.

How are we to work with this shadow material? The psychiatrist Stanislav Grof, with the benefit of his 60 years of experience of HAP states, tells us that the unfolding process is entirely natural, integrative and orientated towards our growth[11]. The shadow encounter of the bad trip is merely a prelude to a rebirth, if the process is properly supported and held. The assumption is that there is an inner intelligence with a benign trajectory, and this trajectory becomes more powerful in the HAP state. The implication is that any material that arises in the psyche will be precisely what is required for the person's move towards wholeness. It is the role of the sitter or facilitator to simply support this natural, unfolding process.

Plato's Cave and the Suntanned Guru

Plato penned his allegory of the cave some 2500 years ago and it remains, for me, the most helpful way of understanding how archetypal energy interacts with our biological nature and the psycho-social conditioning that shapes our conscious experience[12].

Plato asks us to imagine a situation where people are chained in an underground cave. They are facing the back of the cave and their gaze is fixed so they cannot move their heads. They have been there since childhood and know no other reality. There are two sources of light in the cave: one is from the sun outside which filters into the cave, just taking the edge off the darkness; the other source of light is from a fire. In between the fire and the back of the cave, which serves as a viewing screen, there is a walkway where various objects or effigies are paraded. The people parading the objects sometimes talk amongst themselves; the images and sounds are projected onto the back of the cave and the chained people, of course, take these projections to be their primary and sole reality. They think that the shadows are real and that the totality of their perceptual experience emanates from these flickering shadows. How could they know any different, asks Plato?

There are two parts to the story. Firstly, Plato asks us to consider what it would be like if one of the prisoners is set free of his bonds. It would take some courage for this person to leave his peers, to turn away from what is familiar. It would be difficult to get up into a different position, to use unfamiliar muscles and creaky limbs as he turns away from the back of the cave and tentatively starts to explore an unfamiliar environment. The light of the fire and the seepage of daylight from the sun would dazzle him. His senses are over stimulated; it is certainly frightening but also fascinating, it would have that sense of awe that is the hallmark of a numinous experience. Plato suggests that for many of us, this would be intolerable and we would return to where we feel at home, we would go back to the safety of his two-dimensional world.

In the second scenario, we are asked to imagine our explorer, our psychonaut, being taken all the way out of the cave to the sunlight. Of course, he is completely dazzled and his eyes can't make out very much at all. As his eyes become more accustomed, he would gradually be able to make out the shadows cast by the sun first of all, then his vision would discern actual 'things' themselves, three dimensional objects with colour and texture. Eventually he would cast his eyes upwards and would see the heavens, the stars, the moon and the sun. Plato suggests that after a while the man would come to realise the primary importance of the sun, which is responsible for the light, the heat and the energy that allows growth. Indeed, everything flows from the sun; without the sun there is nothing.

Imagine the man going back into the cave, suggests Plato, feeling sorry for those poor people chained up in the dark. They have built up an elaborate value system around the two-dimensional shadows, rewarding and giving status to those who are quickest at recognising shadows and the order in which they follow each other. Do you think, says Plato, that our former prisoner would covet those honours and envy those people who had status and power at the back of the cave? The answer is that he would not, that he would probably put up with anything rather than go back to the value system of the two-dimensional world.

Furthermore, suggests Plato, our man who has been outside and seen the sun needs some time for his eyes to readjust to the gloom of the cave and he has become slow and backward at recognising the shadows. If he had to compete with the prisoners in identifying the shadows wouldn't he make a fool of himself? Wouldn't his comrades pour scorn on him for having come back with his eyes ruined? Wouldn't they be deeply unimpressed by anything that he had to tell them about where he had been and what he had discovered? It is unlikely that they would want to follow in his footsteps and it is unlikely that they would be receptive to his telling them that they are wrong to value the shadows so much, that there may be something deeper and richer.

Does this story ring any bells for us? Plato compares our everyday world to the confinement of the cave. The firelight is the light of the physical world and our normal state of waking consciousness. The chains represent those attachments that hold us back from growth; our anxieties, our addictions, our greed and our mind chatter to name a few. The effigies and the shadows that reflect them represent our conditioning, our language, our psychological and social structures and the hardwire of our nervous systems. They make up Huxley's reducing valve.

The sunlight is entirely different; it represents a more nebulous, non-physical, spiritual ideal. For Plato, the sun was his 'form of the Good', his God term, the pinnacle of the archetypal domain. It could be likened to the

Self archetype or Brahman/Atman. The sun powers the primary objects outside the cave, with all their colour and three dimensional form. This is the numinous, ineffable, archetypal world that is outside the range of our normal experience. The representations of these objects inside the cave are archetypal images, diminished in meaning to a greater or lesser degree. But the sun is always with us in dilute form, it is in the diffuse daylight that percolates into the cave.

We can find tools that help us ascend through the cave, if we wish, perhaps we can even take a look outside. But how does this help us to understand the psychedelic experience. How do archaidelics work their magic?

In microdosing, we could imagine the intensity of the diffuse daylight becoming subtly more intense. The ratio of sunlight to firelight increases and the shadows perhaps become a little sharper, hold a little more vitality. We don't really notice anything but the quality of the light subtly changing and we are enhanced.

In psycholytic doses, we turn away briefly from the flickering shadows at the back of the cave. We are likely to have an encounter with the effigies. Our enhanced perception of the diffuse sunlight may radically alter our perception. The shadows will seem clearer, sharper and we may usefully work on the psychological structures in our own conditioning that constitute our personal shadow.

In psychedelic doses, we may ascend right up through the cave. It may be a sudden rapturous ascent or it may be a more difficult ascent. We may be dazzled; we may bump our heads; we may find ourselves confronting some powerful effigies and their shadows, but then perhaps we enter the territory where the daylight becomes bright and we leave the firelight behind. If we are lucky we may leave the cave altogether, marvel at the primary objects outside and have a glimpse of the sun.

And what of the guru, the man with the supernatural powers who is completely unaffected when he is given high dose LSD? Perhaps the archaidelic drug doesn't make any difference to him because he is at home in the archetypal world and has transcended the limits of space-time. He is already outside the cave – sitting in the sunshine.

CHAPTER 14

The Epilogenic Model

by Dave King

> *Until you make the unconscious conscious,*
> *it will direct your life and you will call it fate.*
> C.G. Jung

The model of epilogenesis describes an enhancement of a person's ability to exercise conscious choice in a physiological or psychological process. This may happen when ordinarily non-conscious material is brought into consciousness. It is a natural and everyday occurrence and can be achieved through biofeedback, meditation, breathing exercise, physical training, and so forth, but under the influence of psychedelics, epilogenesis may come instantly, and unexpectedly. The word epilogenesis refers to the enablement of choice, and comes from the Greek roots *epiloyi* (meaning 'choice, decision, action') and *genesthai* ('to bring into being').

The accessibility of material to conscious attention

Let us imagine that every idea, ever action, every sensation in the body - the constriction of blood vessels, the waves of peristalsis, our childhood memories, our repressed desires, the pulse, the breath, the pain of stubbing your toe – falls somewhere upon a 'spectrum of accessibility to consciousness' (SAC). This is shown in *Figure 1*. At the far right of the SAC we can see the material that is most likely to be conscious during ordinary waking life, such as extreme pain, and loud noises. A little to the left we see the 'threshold of perception' dividing the material that is conscious and the material that is not. Material may cross this threshold into consciousness through attention, and it may fall away from consciousness through

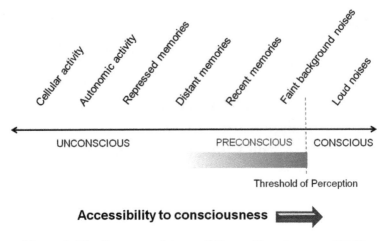

Figure 1. The Spectrum of Accessibility to Consciousness (SAC)

inattention. Two mechanisms operate this: top-down, and bottom-up processing of attention. If you and I were sitting in a café, we might become so absorbed by conversation that we lose awareness of the radio playing softly in the background. If we were to realise this, and make the decision to pay attention to the music, that material would have crossed the threshold of perception by top-down processing. However, if some young miscreant wandered away from his parents and yanked the volume control to maximum, we would achieve awareness (rather suddenly) by bottom-up processing[1].

In 1912, a psychologist by the name of Cheves Perky asked participants in a study to stare at a fixed point on a screen and try to visualise certain objects. Unbeknownst to the participants, images were projected on to the screen so faintly that they were not aware that they were seeing anything. The projected images were too faint to cross the threshold of perception, and were invisible to the conscious mind. But when a horizontal banana was projected and the participants were asked to visualise a banana, their bananas were horizontal too. The invisible images were having an effect.

In Figure 1, the material that approaches the threshold of perception can be thought of as the Freudian preconscious: that which is easily capable of becoming conscious. Neither the conscious nor the preconscious are fixed domains since there is continuous migration of material between them. Let us continue to imagine how items might fall on the SAC: faint background noises such as the radio may lurk just below the threshold, and recent memories a little way behind that. Distant memories may hover somewhere in the murkiness between the preconscious and the unconscious (since the preconscious is that which can readily be made conscious and the unconscious is that which cannot, we might presume that the preconscious fades gradually into the unconscious as material, for whatever reason, becomes less and less accessible). Repressed memories may remain unconscious for the full course of a life, or they may one day migrate upwards. Autonomic physiological activity falls even further down the spectrum – blood rushing through the veins, the processes of digestion, and so on. In the distant reaches of the unconscious, cells grow, fight, protect and communicate with each other with very little likelihood of conscious recognition. Below that , perhaps the body's myriad molecular processes, and beyond that perhaps the atomic.

I think it is fair to say that the vast majority of action in the human system remains unconscious. Indeed, we achieve such little recognition of our own bodies that we fail to notice the growth of tumours, or the build-up of atherosclerosis, or infection from various diseases. Most mothers are not certain of the sex of the child before it is born. In all of these cases, some part of our body is acutely aware of that which we are not, and in the case of illness our immunological selves work tirelessly in attempt of a remedy.

However, we also know that techniques such as biofeedback, breathwork and meditation can help us achieve conscious control over ordinarily non-conscious functions, including heart-rate[2], brain waves (neurofeedback) and blood pressure[3]. Neurofeedback has shown promise as a treatment for addiction[4], depression[5] and epilepsy[6]. The multiple Guinness World Record holder Wim Hof (who in 2007 climbed Everest wearing nothing but shorts, ran a full marathon in the Namib Desert without water in 2011, and who has repeatedly broken the ice endurance record) claims to have learned how to regulate his immune response and body temperature using breath exercises. In 2010, researchers found that he was able to successfully regulate his immune response to exposure of *E. coli*[7], and more recently his methods were used to train study participants to regulate inflammation[8]. These are all examples of non-psychedelic epilogenesis.

Sport and yoga allow us to develop muscle control, and playing the saxophone requires learning to use your breath in new ways. A scholarly lifestyle brings us new ideas, and helps us to reflect upon the world. Psychotherapy allows us to better understand our desires, inner conflicts, and helps relieve pain from traumas. Falling in love is a marvellous aid for developing empathy and understanding. Travellers are often able to absorb languages and cultural beliefs. A visit to the optician may result in markedly improved sight. It is unusual to recall perinatal memories, but some patients may do so under hypnosis[9] or LSD-assisted psychotherapy[10].

What do all of these have in common? They are all examples of conscious-ness expansion: from biofeedback to ball sports, all forms of learning bring new material into conscious attention.

Consciousness expansion & contraction

At this point, it is necessary for us to talk a little about consciousness expansion and contraction, for this will help us bring psychedelics back into the picture. Ralph Metzner offers various analogies for understanding these terms. Firstly, consider the expansion that occurs every morning upon awakening: we first have a dull sense of embodiment as awareness of our physical self returns; then our attention may dedicate itself to reminding you where you are; your mind may next drift to your sleeping partner; and then the building at large, and the town, and all the complex social and professional contexts and responsibilities at hand. This is consciousness expansion. Another analogy that Metzner uses is watching TV: to focus on one character is contractive relative to the contemplation of the whole television program, and that too is contractive relative to the recognition of the television itself, and the room in which you're sitting, and so forth.

But *what is expanding*? What is it expanding into? An LSD trip may very well be an expanded state of consciousness, but what about the tripper with the awe-filled eyes who stares intently at his fingerprints? What about the poor fellow having a mushroom-induced panic attack? How can an experience be both expansive and contractive at the same time? And does expansion always come at the cost of contraction elsewhere? Stan Grof's patients lay on couches with facemasks, their minds far away in the vision-ary realms of archetypes and dreams – expansive, surely, but at the cost of contraction in the here-and-now physical domains of the room, just as the studious computer programmer jumps when you tap him on the shoulder. And, conversely, the blear-eyed bed bug of Metzner's first analogy - weren't they suffering a contraction of consciousness in whatever domain dreams are supposed to arise from?

Metzner[11] identifies four domains into and from which consciousness may expand or contract:

Ideas, thoughts and cognitive processes;
Visual images (plus sounds, smells, tastes, etc.);
Emotions, affects and feelings;
Body sensations (tactile, kinaesthetic, thermal, etc.)

Although he does not specify this, I think it is clear that these are best thought of as the domains usually accessible during waking consciousness.

It does not seem likely that this is the end of it. For instance, from which of these four domains do we suppose out-of-body experiences, K-holes, salvia-induced 'alternate realities', death and rebirth experiences, dreams, psychedelic visions, McKenna's self-transforming machine elves, spontaneous mystical experiences and parapsychological phenomena arise?

Grof[12] proposes an additional two domains:

Experiences occurring in psychedelic and holotropic sessions cannot be described in terms of the narrow and superficial conceptual model used in academic psychiatry and psychology, which is limited to biology, postnatal biography and the Freudian individual unconscious. Deep experiential work requires a vastly extended cartography of the psyche that includes important domains uncharted by traditional science. My own version of such a model includes two additional levels of the psyche, for which I use the terms perinatal and transpersonal.

Now, can we feel comfortable that we have defined these six domains as the source of all human experience? Do we need to add more? I think that depends on whether you are, at heart, a lumper or a splitter, since the precise distinctions between these domains may be difficult. Ana Maqueda, founder of the salvia research organisation *Xka Pastora*, described to me how many salvia users describe their experiences in terms of vivid 'alternate realities'. Let's think about the other highly-specific psychedelic states: DMT entities, K-holes, ibogaine ancestral underworlds, etc. Do these all herald from the same domain? Perhaps Grof's cartography is reflective of the fact that he is therapeutically familiar with LSD. Yet, we continue to see new drugs all the time that affect consciousness in new ways. Are these different experiences all manifestations of the same material with different idiosyncrasies, expectations and cultural viewpoints, or are we witnessing material from conceptually distinct realms? If the latter, how many are there? How many stations can the radio pick up? How big is the job market for novel psychedelics?

Perhaps it doesn't matter. Why is it important to identify the source domains of an experience? One way or another, an experience is always real – we know this because *you had the experience*. So why bother talking about domains?

Well, let us consider two situations. In the first, a patient has a powerful experience which s/he believes to be a repressed memory. It is quite common to recover repressed memories – as Grof writes: '*Repressed unconscious material, including early childhood memories, becomes easily available* [during an LSD experience] '[13]. However, research shows that in some cases, uncovered memories turn out to be false[14]. It will matter a great deal whether the experience has come from a vault of repressed trau-matic material or from that illusive realm 'the imagination'. Consider near-death experiences: is the light at the end of the tunnel the result of experience within an ordinarily inaccessible spiritual domain, or is it just tunnel vision as a result of reduced blood flow to the eyes – i.e. from ordinary sense domains? The on-going debate about the ontology of DMT beings simply comes down to a debate over their source-domain: are they expressions of your own personality, archetypal beings, or independent sentient entities?

With this brief discussion of domains out of the way, let us return to consciousness expansion. I propose that there are at least four ways of looking at consciousness expansion:

Acute expansion: the immediate state of attentive focus described in Metzner's TV analogy. This can be symbolised on the SAC by increas-ing the permeability of the threshold of perception, or by moving it fur-ther into the preconscious.

Episodic expansion: characterised by a period in which (a) the potential for acute expansion is heightened, or (b) which significantly facilitates transference of new material into consciousness. This can be symbol-ised on the SAC by expanding the preconscious further into the uncon-scious.

Chronic expansion: a permanent unlocking of material which can read-ily be made conscious. This is the form of expansion associated with most forms of learning. This can be symbolised on the SAC by noting the migration of material toward consciousness.

Parallel expansion: in which access to domains is locked and unlocked. Since the SAC may be drawn from any available domain, parallel expansion adds or removes material to/from the spectrum. In Metzner's TV analogy, parallel expansion is represented by changing the channel.

With this proposal, we are able to answer our earlier questions:

'What is expanding? What is it expanding into?' In acute expansion, the 'conscious' area on the SAC expands into the 'preconscious'; in epi-sodic expansion, the 'preconscious' expands into the 'unconscious'; in par-allel expansion, consciousness migrates between domains of awareness – such as falling asleep or waking up. *'How can a state of mind be simultaneously contractive and expansive?'* Our poor fellow having a mushroom-induced panic attack is experiencing acute contraction in a period of episodic expansion.

According to a 2014 Salon article, it was Zen priest Kokyo Henkel who first said that spiritual development is a mountain, and that psychedelics give you a brief helicopter ride to the top. It is the advantage of long-term spiritual techniques to unlock chronic expansion.

Psychedelic action

The action of psychedelics is rather complicated, but two particular features may be described as follows:

Psychedelics cause a non-specific migration of material into conscious awareness
(opening the reducing valve).

Although the effect of psychedelics on unconscious material is considered non-specific, researchers and users have long been aware of factors that contribute to the content of the experience. The established notions of *set* – which refers to material from the personal, internal domains – and *setting* – which refers to material from the public domains – describe the primary factors that affect the probability of material becoming conscious[15]. If a patient has a psychedelic experience in the context of focused, on-going psychotherapy, there is a good probability that the material made conscious will be pertinent, but the less preparation and expectation there is for a psychedelic experience, the broader the scope for material able to be transferred – a potentially dangerous situation. Grof comments:

[Psychedelics] *increase the energetic niveau in the psyche and body which leads to manifestation of otherwise latent psychological processes*[16]

It is necessary to structure and approach the experience in a specific way to make the emergence of unconscious material therapeutic rather than destructive[17]

Psychedelics make accessible domains of awareness that cannot ordinarily be reached (by most people) without mind-manifesting techniques (pharmacological or otherwise). As the first line in Leary & Metzner's *The Psychedelic Experience* says: '*A psychedelic experience is a journey to new realms of consciousness*[18]'.

Choice & epilogenesis

Whether or not it is ultimately illusory, choice is a word for describing decisions that are made with conscious direction. I may decide to wave to a friend, but if I instinctively gesticulate while giving a lecture, I am moving my arm without thought. If I use a skipping rope, I am choosing to jump. If someone frightens me, I jump without choice. The further down on the SAC the process, the less control can be exercised with regard to it. For instance, breathing is ordinarily automatic, but we can all quite easily bring it into consciousness and change the way we breathe. Digestion, on the other hand, falls much further down the spectrum and very little choice can be exercised. When an ordinarily unconscious cognitive or physical process is transferred into consciousness, either through practice or non-specific psychedelic migration, it may benefit (or suffer) from being newly amenable to conscious interference.

Some of the various reported applications of psychedelic consciousness include the treatment of addictions[19,20,21], compulsive behaviours[22], allergies and autoimmune disorders[23], and negative behavioural patterns. What do these things have in common? They all seem to involve some sort of process that is not ordinarily amenable to conscious attention. Psychedelics may help because the migration of material into consciousness – either accidentally or with forethought – may be pertinent to these ordinarily non-conscious processes, just as many of these problems have been successfully treated with biofeedback-based epilogenesis.

Consider the report below of Andrew Weil, Professor of Medicine, Public Health and Integrative Rheumatology at the University of Arizona, in which an episode of psychedelic consciousness occasioned by LSD led to an epilogenic remission of a cat allergy:

> I was very allergic as a kid, in all sorts of ways. I had hay fever, I got hives in response to various things. One of the allergies I had was to cats: whenever a cat got near me my eyes would itch, my nose would run; if I touched the cat this would get much worse and if the cat licked me I would break out in hives... so I had a mindset that I was allergic to cats and didn't want them in my presence... there was a deep, ingrained defensiveness in my interactions with cats. One day, when I was twenty-eight, I took LSD with some friends. I was in a terrific space, the world was magical, everything was wonderful, and into this scene a cat bounded and jumped in my lap. I had a split second of the habitual reaction and suddenly I decided this was silly, why did I have to do this? So I started petting the cat, I started playing with the cat, I had no reaction. I haven't had a reaction to a cat since, and that was almost forty years ago[24]

Weil describes how his allergic response was 'deep' and 'ingrained', from which we can assume that it, like most allergies, was unconscious. During the LSD experience he 'suddenly decided' to react differently, which indicates that he had become conscious of the process and was able to exercise choice where previously he had none.

Choice is not necessarily a useful thing to have too much of. In his book *Confessions of a Romantic Reductionist*, the neuroscientist Christof Koch explains that a cunning golfer can put a competitor off their shot by bringing their attention to their posture or position. This attention makes the player acutely aware of his stance on his next shot, and procedural memory is not permitted to do its job. Likewise, when I have given this talk in Canterbury and Berlin, I asked the audience if they had ever experienced, during a state of psychedelic consciousness, confusion resulting from not being able to perform ordinarily automatic actions such as walking, talking, lifting a cup of water, or maintaining balance. I then requested that they keep their hands up if they felt that, at least on one occasion, this was because they had to really figure out and consciously direct themselves to perform an action that they could usually do without thinking. Somewhere between one-half and two-thirds of the audience held their hands in the air.

Predictions

Psychedelic consciousness may have therapeutic potential in conditions where the opposite of epilogenesis has occurred, and previously conscious processes have become unconscious. These situations include incontinence and loss of motor control in the elderly; loss of motor control following a stroke or brain injury; and spasticity. Moreover, there may be advantages to researching the possibility of psychedelically-assisted self-diagnostics. We know that in a psychotherapeutic setting we can make the subject of psychedelic material highly specific. If researchers supervised a series of clinical LSD sessions as part of a three month physiology, pathology and immunology course, with the specific intention of performing self-diagnostics, could we teach people how to scan their own bodies for tumours, inflammation and disease?

Conclusions

I present the following argument:

We do not ordinarily have conscious awareness of most of the processes of body or mind. With psychedelics, and other practices, we can expand consciousness within and between domains of awareness, and may as a result achieve conscious awareness of ordinarily non-conscious processes.

On some occasions, this enhanced awareness may facilitate conscious manipulation of ordinarily-inaccessible processes: this is *epilogenesis*. Epilogenesis may help us understand the broad applications of psychedelic consciousness, and may help encourage preparation and integration.

It should be clear that there is no such thing as an epilogen except in reference to a particular state of consciousness. It is misleading to suggest that any particular compound is an epilogen unconditionally, but it is acceptable to state that 'the subject had an episode of epilogenic consciousness in which X was the epilogen'.

The critic may suggest that one has no choice over what one experiences during psychedelic consciousness, and that it is a fundamentally passive process. This may be so, but epilogenesis does not explain what psychedelic consciousness is; it simply offers a description of one possible, perhaps therapeutic side-effect.

CHAPTER 15

Femtheogens
The Synergy of Sacred Spheres

by Maria Papaspyrou

> *Taking the next evolutionary step toward the Archaic Revival, the*
> *rebirth of the Goddess, and the ending of profane history will require*
> *an agenda that includes the notion of our reinvolvement with and the*
> *emergence of the vegetable mind.*
>
> Terence McKenna

There appears to be a recent proliferation of psychedelic neologisms. This seems to correlate with 'psychedelic culture' embracing, in the last decade, a new sense of agency, which has been based on an amplified resurgence of theoretical and research-based explorations. The emergent lexical expansions create welcomed openings, as each new word unravels potential aspects of the multiplicity of the psychedelic experience.

The word I have been exploring is 'femtheogens', a compound word of 'feminine' and 'entheogens'. Entheogens is yet another compound word made up from 'entheo' and 'genesis' that refers to the mystical and sacred properties of the psychedelic experience. Femtheogens, through its roots in 'entheogens', refers to the feminised sacredness of the experiences such substances can induce. It refers to the capacity of the entheogenic experience to revive the broken sacred feminine, and filter its essence through to us. This capacity is enhanced by the strong connections between the archetypal feminine and the entheogenic experience. The two share qualities that can heal, transform, and support the expansion of our consciousness. These qualities are also major points of suppression for both, as they run counter to our western mindset and emergent social paradigms.

In the Garden of Eden, Eve took a bite from the apple of the Sacred Tree of Knowledge. This was a mythos that repressed both the feminine, and expanded awareness, into sin within our consciousness, merging them with the shadow side. Mythologically and symbolically, this was the onset point of ego development for our species. To leave the Garden was to gain self-awareness, up until that point we lived in the unconscious Eden. Today, in our predominantly ego driven reality, we still keep femtheogenic consciousness in exile, we systematically maintain its inferiority, and we remain suspicious of its depth and potential. The feminine and entheogens have been suppressed because their force and energy could not be assimilated by our species. We have distorted both to a diabolical form and seen them as dangerous and seductive forces.

Archetypal Feminine Realms

In trying to reveal some of the feminine nature and quality, I will be focusing on the archetypal feminine. Archetypes are collective psychic entities, loaded symbols and metaphors, that mediate between unconscious depths and consciousness. As an archetype the feminine is always and ever present, inhabiting the depths of our collective unconscious where the archetypes reside, from where she addresses us both individually and collectively. In our collective disconnection from the archetypal feminine voice and essence, we have lost our ability to integrate her energies and offerings. But her essence is relevant to all of us, because the feminine is an elemental pattern we all carry within ourselves, whether we are a man or women. And she is also relevant to everything around us, because the feminine is the one half of the Divine Androgyne, which is the deepest archetype that permeates all of creation.

Gareth Hill[1] is a Jungian analyst who has explored the intrapsychic aspects of gender. He has divided the feminine in her static and her dynamic aspect, mapping out the deepest and most essential qualities of the feminine force.

The 'static feminine'[2] is connected to motherhood and nourishment, holding deep primal secrets of creation within her body. She can conceive the potential of life and give birth to it, participating in the great mystery of manifesting a soul into material life[3]. In that mystery, the feminine participates in the forces of creation and regeneration. It is this feminine link to regeneration that makes her central to our collective healing process. Woman magic and earth magic are linked; they both create and nourish life[4]. The static feminine is impersonal like nature, and serves the collective goals of life on earth, which is species preservation and survival. For our early ancestors, the feminine link with nature was at first a point of worship, until man tried to control, manipulate, and suppress the force, creating a deep imbalance in his relationship with it.

The 'dynamic feminine'[5] is represented by a surrendering watery flow "towards the new, the non-rational, and the playful"[6]. She is spontaneous, responsive, intuitive, and forms according to what fate brings her way. She receives her wisdom by engaging with direct experience, and is receptive to knowledge that belongs to the deep inner worlds. She opens us to sublime encounters, and owns the spaces of spontaneous realisation. She is connected to the creative and regenerative aspects of chaos, and supports the expansive creative synthesis of new possibilities and subsequent evolution. The dynamic feminine represents spaces that can be fascinating and ecstatic as well as terrifying and disorienting, and these are watery transient spaces that as a society we have learnt to resist.

In today's society, the Goddess has lost her lineage and her priestesses. In the absence of her guides, she meets us in the land of the unconscious[7] and the realms of altered consciousness, where her feminine work can go on undisturbed. She communicates with us through the archaic symbolic language of dreams and imagination. In our western world we focus on language, which is the ordered and rational container of experience, a masculine principle. The realms beyond that space belong to the feminine, and there we meet that which is beyond words.

The myths and words we hold the feminine in, control her essence and energies. By holding the feminine in words like irrational, emotional, hysterical, subjective, chaotic, etc. we have linked her with energies that our societies have always feared and tried to control. However, the word 'feminine' refers to the Soul[8]. It is a reference to the cosmic thread that connects us to each other and to the rest of creation. It acknowledges our interconnectedness and place within a cosmic sacred order, linking us to life and the divine.

Femtheogenic Consciousness

I have called it femtheogenic consciousness because how we relate to the points below can have a profound effect on how we experience and relate to the world around us, and in effect recalibrate our moral compass. But for that to happen, we must resurrect the true and deeper essence of both the feminine and entheogens, from the tenebrous depths of our unconscious, where both have been repressed by patriarchy.

One of the major insights femtheogenic consciousness opens us up to is the awareness of connectedness and oneness. Our illusion of separateness has for centuries alienated us from earth, each other, and the deepest nature of our own selves. In our fragmented state we have disconnected man from nature. We have imposed our hierarchical relational structures on our desacralized world, and placed our species in the dominator's position. And from that narcissistic bubble, all we can recognise in the mirrors of the world around us is ourselves[9], and our own needs. We have assumed that our needs entitle us to control and manipulate all natural resources for our own advantage, and we have created a crisis that is environmental, social, and spiritual.

Femtheogenic consciousness operates in the spheres of oneness. This oneness is a spiritual connection that reveals the reflections we emit to each other. We are all mirrors of our shared humanity, and we all hold each other within ourselves. This oneness is not only a metaphysical idea[10]. It is the oneness that chaos theorists have called the butterfly effect, where a butterfly flaps its wings on one continent and causes a hurricane, weeks later, on another continent. This is the oneness of cause and effect, a very direct way of experiencing the world around us. The feminine consciousness is by nature aware that everything is connected. This is a knowledge the feminine has always carried in her body's centre of creation, where all life emerges and regenerates from. Similarly, in the infinite realms of entheogenic channels, we can witness the threads of our interconnectedness and interdependence. Here we encounter the pulsating presence of Indra's net, and meet the potential of reawakening our links with each other, nature, the divine, and ultimately ourselves. The invisible space of singularity that femtheogenic consciousness reveals to us contains Eros at its core. To recognise its presence, is to awaken to the most powerful force in the universe.

The next femtheogenic consciousness link is boundary-dissolving experiences. Our societies are based on divisive boundaries that maintain the illusion of our separateness, and the ultimate and most dreaded boundary to cross is the dissolution of the ego. The ego has been a big part of our evolution, and as a concept in itself it can have many useful functions, what is dysfunctional is our need to hold on to it. The ego needs to undergo many deaths if we are to transform into a more authentic version of ourselves. We need to peel through the layers to reach through to the core of who we really are. The essence of feminine consciousness is based on the elementary feminine experience of boundary dissolution, motherhood, where the 'Other' is contained within oneself. That symbiotic bond is not merely a physical one as it extends way beyond the physical birthing process. Entheogenic experiences are also, by their very nature, based on the dissolution of boundaries on various levels. In these realms, the divisive lines between past, present, and future, us and Other, conscious and unconscious, masculine and feminine, dissolve, and that is the most threatening aspect of entheogenic consciousness for both individuals and the general status quo[11]. Both the Great Goddess and entheogenic journeys, deliver us to a point where in order to evolve, we need to transcend our boundaries, and release ourselves from the ego-driven mirage of our delicate reality.

The next femtheogenic consciousness link relates to chaos. We have battled for generations to tame chaos because we have perceived it to be one of our greatest survival threats. It hasn't always been like that, the early Gnostics and Alchemists recognised chaos as a vital element of the creative process of transformation. Today we relate to chaos as a state of disintegration, rather than a stage of transformation. We have failed to acknowledge the inherent order it contains because its nature is creative rather than linear, it is not to be imposed, it is to emerge[12]. In its field resides the rhythms of matter and the deeper wisdom of the creative process. For our ancestors the Goddess was linked with nature, and as they gradually viewed nature as a chaotic force that needed to be controlled, they reflected that onto the feminine, installing our unconscious collective link between the Feminine and chaos. But the archetypal feminine, in its 'dynamic' aspect, has a creative link with chaos, and that is a link with the transformative and regenerative aspects of chaos. Entheogenic journeys embrace chaos and its transformative potential, and teach us it is a valued stage in our unfolding process of individuation. During a deep entheogenic journey we are taken apart and then put back together. Chaos gives birth to a new order that is of greater complexity than before, a step further on our evolutionary journey. A big part of what drove our connection with nature, the Goddess, and entheogens underground is our collective difficulty to be with chaos, and femtheogenic consciousness holds the potential of reviving that relationship in a meaningful way.

The next femtheogenic link relates to the vital cycles of life, death, and rebirth. For our early ancestors, the feminine powers of fertility and birth were a reflection of cosmic regeneration. Nature's wisdom taught them that death is a stage of regeneration rather than an end in itself. Today we relate to death with dread, unable to face its vital essence and relate to it on a deeper level, and we are immersed in a collective and all encompassing denial of death. The Goddess Kali is a powerful archetypal feminine symbol of the regenerative wisdom. In Kali's terms the Goddess who gives life is the Goddess who takes life; creation gives place to destruction, destruction that is in service to life gives place to creation, a ceaseless movement that is indifferent to our ego's demands for survival[13]. According to C. G. Jung, "the descent into the depths always seems to precede the ascent"[14]. We can only recover our inner gifts and treasures by meeting the dark side of the archetypal feminine; the devourer and the transformer. Similarly, the most potent entheogenic experiences that people report, with the greatest and most profound changes, are journeys within a supportive set and setting, unfolding into the ultimate spiritual experience of ego-death. Femtheogenic consciousness allows us to flee our ego, if only for a second, and receive the wisdom that necessitates and even welcomes death. That is not to negate the painful experience of crossing the transition portals of change, death, and loss. That is to also access the femtheogenic wisdom that teaches us that it is the ego that grieves. On a soul level things are different, because our souls know that every end is a drop in a vast ocean[15].

Time is a major symbol in our society that we have learned to treat as a fixed and static construct. But the feminine rhythms of regeneration reveal timelessness. The archetypal Goddess of birth contains a soul that moves through various birth canals. She participates in a mystery that intersects time. Entheogenic spaces also hold timelessness, revealing to us within a journey mysteries that defy our ordinary experiential parameters and boundaries, allowing us to move through past, present, and future in extraordinary ways. Through femtheogenic consciousness we come to witness and experience a very different sense of time.

The next femtheogenic link is creativity. Patriarchy has suppressed our creative forces by focusing on the mind and the logic. But femtheogenic consciousness supports the creative dimension of our evolution. The feminine is the creative matrix of life for our species. She resonates with the patterns that belong to creation. The archetypal feminine is also linked to experience, immersion, and surrender; yielding and responsive she channels the energies of imagination. Entheogenic journeys are highly creative spaces. They 'speak' to us through symbols, images, and feeling states that are carried forward by visions. These openings create metaphors that connect us to that which is beyond words or beyond immediate perception. These are the same spaces that the artists, visionaries, mystics, and shamans, navigate and draw their inspiration and wisdom from. But our societies have not acknowledged the creative and ultimately healing potential of these spaces, and we only relate to them as chaotic, destructive, and dangerous states.

Femtheogenic consciousness carries a particular kind of wisdom that our culture has long neglected and avoided. Our cultural estrangement from feminine and entheogenic sources of intelligence has deprived us from knowledge that penetrates deep within the reaches of the invisible. Femtheogenic knowing is intuitive, non-linear, and informed by the creative source. It has the potency to reveal to us the invisible, and that includes the invisible corners of our psyche. This is where our shadow lives. Claiming our shadow and its darkness helps us cultivate compassion for ourselves, and in reflection for others. This is where we encounter the limitations of our human nature and where the heart works on forgiveness. The mind carries the logic while the heart carries the wisdom. In this deeply reflective space dualities fall through, here we can heal the psychic divides we have succumbed to, and invoke the restorative inner forces of integration.

Femtheogenic consciousness opens us up to spontaneous, instinctual, and authentic ways of living. In trying to shield ourselves from our impermanence and lack of control, we have learned to perceive the world and reality as concrete. This concreteness offers us a 'safety', but it can also lead to staleness, and deadness, which is ironically the very thing our egos are trying to avoid. We operate from a state of doing unable to tolerate a state of being. Femtheogenic consciousness embraces change and impermanence, aware that this is the foundational basis of evolutionary drives. The true essence of the feminine is not bounded by rules, or order. She exists in a freedom that is full of potential. She is not identified with the social personas that we are predestined to hold onto in our patriarchal society; she is receptive to experience with a sense of self that is expansive. Entheogens too, by dissolving our egos, allow us to die and be reborn infinite times within the space of a few hours, shaking away our social masks and helping us question the unquestionable. In these spaces we can encounter wholeness, and a natural intelligence that is buried deeply within us. The dissolution of our personas facilitates the ultimate goal of development, individuation, the growth into one's true self and potential. Who we become under the guidance of femtheogenic consciousness can be far wider and broader than what the stagnant social matrix allows us to ever imagine.

The final femtheogenic link I will explore is the unconscious. The unconscious is an entity that is not containable in a rational system of causality. In the symbolic world of Jungian analytical psychology, consciousness is carried by the masculine while the unconscious is the terrain of the feminine. And indeed this is where the feminine and entheogenic experiences have been relegated to by society, to the collective unconscious depths. It is the dynamic feminine that is linked to the invisible symbolic spaces of our psyche, and she communicates these spaces into our consciousness through imagination and altered states of consciousness. Entheogenic journeys raise unconscious material into consciousness, allowing us to access our undercurrent realms. Femtheogenic openings to these deep spaces can create the potential for our conscious and unconscious selves to meet and integrate, paving the way for our psychological journey towards wholeness.

The War on Femtheogenic Consciousness

Patriarchy is a paranoid state of consciousness that tries to suppress any potential for power or anything that threatens its structures, and has actively waged a war against both the feminine and entheogens. Patriarchy is a power system that breeds unjust hierarchical power relations. It suppresses any true form of individualism, and teaches us to think that our value as a person is linked to our position in its structures. We adopt its worldview, wear our personas, and come to believe that we actually are what we appear to be.

Today, patriarchy's attack on the feminine is a collective responsibility. We are all part of a culture that attacks nature and the feminine in all of us. We all have to delve deep within ourselves and recognise where we have played our own part in her oppression and betrayed her essence. In our masculine culture we have suppressed the feminine force. We have lost our knowledge and connection to her ancient mystery traditions, and have denied her wisdom in the rational and scientific world we have created and surrounded ourselves with. By dissecting the essence of the feminine and throwing its essential elemental patterns away, we have deprived ourselves from the potential of connecting with the feminine wholeness, the unifying principle of creation. Men have also been wounded and alienated from patriarchy's attacks on the feminine. The devaluing of the feminine has damaged the feminine within men, because we all hold a part of that archetype in our psychic depths. Patriarchy has also alienated men from the feminine outside themselves, by splitting them between their need to idealise the feminine and their fearful need to dominate and control her[16].

Patriarchy has also been in conflict with entheogens. Patriarchy has traditionally favoured substances that maintain boundaries, create a mindless state, and support the status quo[17]. Terence McKenna has written about the links between the ban of entheogens and the suppression of the sacred feminine, and the rise of patriarchy[18]. For McKenna, through the war on femtheogens, transcendental experiences were replaced by "dogma, priest craft, patriarchy, warfare, and eventually "rational and scientific" or dominator values"[19]. Entheogenic experiences deliver us to the land of ambiguity, helping us question what it all means and why things are as they are, allowing us to consider alternative possibilities that are usually more planet and people friendly. They cut through our cultural conditioning and offer us a wider lens to examine what we call 'reality', that is beyond our dominant cultural paradigms. They catalyse imagination and the expansion of our consciousness. And very importantly, they reawaken and unify the fractured feminine, and filter her essence through to us, reviving and transmitting her essential regenerative and restorative energies. It is no coincidence that during the psychedelic wave of the 1950s and 60s, and under the influence of psychedelic expansions, all forms of oppression were questioned. It was the time the ecological, anti-war, and feminist movements emerged, amongst others, seeds that are still growing today. Entheogenic experiences make the maintenance of rigid hierarchies unsustainable and that poses a major threat to patriarchy[20]. Patriarchy, in response to that threat, has done a very good job at making us believe that the use of psychedelics is an immoral and antisocial threat, and it has validated the criminal persecution of cognitive liberty, which is the freedom to alter or enhance one's consciousness.

As Within, So Without; As above, So below

The recovery of the femtheogenic energy is integral for reviving the political, social, economic, and spiritual desolation we are currently facing.

On an individual level, our levels of unhappiness are soaring, and our narcissistic worldview leaves us powerless, paranoid, and with low self-esteem. We have neglected our hearts and deprived ourselves from the sanctuary of community and relationships. We instead live our lives increasingly more from cyber space where our false selves thrive, and we disconnect further away from any true knowledge of ourselves. In our internal and external state of alienation we give in more and more to diseases of the mind and the body.

But nothing exists in isolation, as femtheogenic consciousness knows and teaches us all too well. The individual psyche is a reflection and a microcosm of the cultural macrocosm, and our individual crisis translates to a horrifying social crisis.

The zeitgeist of our desacralized secular society is consumerism and materialism, which we refuse to moderate[21]. Our post-modern deities have taken monetary forms. In our target driven societies we have forgotten how to care for each other and ourselves. We have forgotten how to support and honour our elders, and have abandoned our youths to the mercy of ruthless media that shrink their souls, and neglect the development of their highest potential. In the meantime, we are busy waging wars of ideology, religion, and race[22]. In our dominator, hierarchical societies we have lost sight of the importance of equality and partnership. We are facing overpopulation and tragic issues such as hunger, water shortages, sanitation, and the spread of infectious diseases in various parts of our world, that are not being effectively addressed.

Our individual and social crisis also extends to the ecology around us. We have ravaged our rainforests, we have overfished and depleted our seas, we have contaminated our rivers, we have excavated our mountains, and our ever-increasing demands for food and technology are depleting earth's vital resources. Our exploitation of earth and its resources is amounting to ecocide, as we irreversibly disrupt ecosystems that species depend on. Our ecocidal tendencies are also linked to our genocidal tendencies, as we are waging wars on the basis of diminishing resources[23].

The moment of crisis activates the potential for deep transformation. All birthing initiates in the darkness. We have to face our shadows before the "old solidified ego boundaries can be shattered"[24], and through the cracks the possibility of something new can emerge. The process of transformation is based on the tension of opposites, and it feels like we are treading a very thin line[25]. On the one side lies the potential of evolution, through the integration of powerful forces. On the other side lies the danger of social disintegration and regression into the worst possible scenarios of human nature. Dangerous reactionary forces awake during the time of rebirth with the capacity to threaten our visions[26] and reassert the existing status quo.

Invoking archaic vestiges: Anima Mundi

At the dawn of human consciousness, our early ancestors lived in a symbiotic relationship with nature. In their concrete and magical thinking, they created mythologies where nature was personified through the Great Mother, powerful and vital in the threading of life and death. This image was one of our earliest collective blueprints on the nature of God. When the Sun God replaced the Earth Goddess, we lost that connection to nature and became alienated from the most profound source of life and wisdom. That divine source of creation, the soul of the world, was once known as anima mundi. Anima mundi was the spirit that resides within the centre of every living thing and held the knowledge that there is consciousness within matter[27]. Our ancestors used sacred ritual to activate this light of the world soul, invoking a communion with creation, where light spoke to light.

In our current western cosmological framework we relate to anima mundi only as a concept as we no longer live a life that is aligned to its principles. We have desacralized nature and forgotten that the world is alive. We no longer relate to this light within nature or within ourselves. We have disconnected from our imaginative and intuitive potential, and we have lost touch with the magic stuff.

Meditations, mantras, breathing exercises, entheogens, can all activate aspects of the inner technology of our species, and belong to the magical side of our human experience[28]. They return us to an embodied wisdom and transform our ego consciousness to a soul consciousness. A connection with anima mundi, the world soul, can bring us back into connection with our own soul.

Mythopoetic Metamorphosis

The ultimate developmental goal in Jungian psychology is individuation; the growth into one's full potential. We cannot individuate unless we integrate our shadow material. Patriarchy has repressed the feminine and its values in our collective shadow, and until we retrieve and integrate her essence in our psychic development, we will continue to act out our neurotic fantasies, and endanger our survival on this planet. We are also being called to retrieve our archaic intelligence, and cultivate a direct experience and relationship with 'Mind at Large', through spiritual practices and/or entheogenic experiences.

As a species we receive powerful directional energies from language, myths, symbols and metaphors, cultural memes, and ideas. Our narrative worlds can shape and form our consciousness and evolutionary expansions. There has been a lot of talk about the return of the divine feminine. The return of the divine feminine is essentially a new mythology for challenging the existing patriarchal structures and for the expansion of our consciousness. It speaks of a change in our attitude towards nature, our planet, and our own bodies. To release the Goddess is to cultivate a relationship to the deep cosmic source of our psychic lives and come to care for all creation[29]. The divine feminine asks us to transcend our divisive ideologies, to hold a responsible presence on this planet, and to foster emotional intelligence for the generations that are to come.

The masculine and the feminine are the fundamental archetypal energies of life that make up the entire universe. They are complementary and compensating forces. We are being called to create new mythologies that integrate the alchemical union of the lunar feminine wisdom with the solar masculine consciousness. The archetypal union of the masculine and the feminine principles holds the promise of wholeness. A healthy future needs to be balanced by the Divine Androgyne.

What we today call western civilisation has evolved out of the dissociation between man and nature. This dissociation has been mirrored in our separation of matter and spirit, soul and body, thinking and feeling, reason and instinct, masculine and feminine, life and death. In our dualistic worldview we have lost sight of the wholeness and totality such tensions hold.

Our future potential depends on being able to embrace the whole spectrum of such continuums.

Evolution for our species at this point is no longer a matter of physicality; it is now a matter of interiority[30]. We need to go within and discover who we really are away from the social personas we have adapted to. This is not just about having insights, change means change. We may have to die to our jobs, our relationships, our faiths, our false selves, and everything that no longer serves the freedom of our deepest nature. Every one of these deaths is a sacred initiation towards the emergence of our true self. To enter the core is to awaken the light that resides within the core of every living thing; to enter the core is to invoke the anima mundi.

The feminine, entheogens, and nature, can only be liberated after social revolution results in structural change. Patriarchy as a system needs to be challenged. Nations around the world are trying to shed away the politically expired systems and their archaic socio-political complexes. On an individual and a collective level we are seeking greater truth and freedom. We are one step away from assuming responsibility and participation, which is where our true freedom lies. For all these energies to transform we need the strong container of the Goddess. And entheogens are a powerful channel of the feminine voice and essence. They bring us into alignment with the sacred core and remind us of the divine purpose of being alive.

The revival of femtheogenic consciousness can support the emergence of a planetary consciousness. Our crisis is a crisis of consciousness. The world's wounds and imbalances are a reflection of our own wounds and imbalances[31]; first we have to rescue our own souls. That is how we participate in the mystery of oneness.

When sentient matter becomes a vessel for the enormity of the soul, we can transcend the alienated and fragmented levels of consciousness our one-sided materiality bounds us to. "A world that is not connected to the soul cannot heal"[32]. Femtheogenic consciousness can guide us in a creative relationship towards our deepest Self, and its myriad outward reflection.

CHAPTER 16

Re-Habituating Cognition
An Interview with former LSD Chemist Casey Hardison

questions by Robert Dickins

One carries freedom inside oneself, a man with a good mind will realise his potential in any regime...He does not pass through the regimes, they pass through him, barely leaving a trace.
- Ernst Jünger, Aladdin's Problem

Everybody who reasons carefully about something is making a contribution to the knowledge of what happens when you think about something.
- Richard Feymnan, The Relation of Mathematics and Physics

PPUK: *Hi Casey, thanks very much for answering some of our questions and, more importantly, blessings and congratulations on your recent release from Her Majesty's pleasure. In February 2004, you were arrested on suspicion of manufacturing a number of entheogens such as LSD, DMT, and 2-CB. How did the arrest go down, and what was going through your mind?*

Casey Hardison: Well, I was high at the time, on LSD and the love of life, and I was downstairs in the Sanctuary Cafe in Brighton/Hove, watching and recording an absolutely lovely voice: Kat Drake. This man in plain clothes walks up to me, way too straight for the 'sanctuary' I was allegedly in; and he, being Detective Sargent Pike of the Sussex Police, with his hand on my upper arm, says to me something to the effect of: 'Mr Hardison, Mr Casey Hardison'. Realizing I was busted so few words into his sentence, DS Pike continued, 'I would like to arrest you on the suspicion of manufacturing controlled drugs'. I said, 'OK, how do you want to do this?' DS Pike said, 'As calmly as possible'. I replied, 'Right on, me too'. You see, he was trying to bust an acid chemist and I was standing in a room full of hippies who didn't notice a thing was going on. My friend Pete just remembers I was there and then I wasn't.

'As part of doing this,' I said to Pike, 'I have a request'. He said 'Go ahead'. As I was surrounded by my stills and video cameras, plus microphones and other necessary miscellany, I prefaced my request by paraphrasing a dead president: 'Since Government is instituted to protect property of every sort, and as you are a member of the government, I request that you protect my property'. Pike then asked me to identify my property and quietly called for the assistance of another plainclothes Officer who set about gathering my property to my satisfaction. (Curiously, all these items were later returned and not subject to confiscation orders.)

Two or three minutes later, after policing my property peacefully, in a room full of hippies who take no notice, Pike escorts me up the stairs and out the door, and hands me over to Detective Constable Cutriss, who then helps me into a paper suit as though touching me too much might get them high. Did they learn this from Operation Julie? Later I would find out that this learning was not that deep or sophisticated. After DC Cutriss gets me into the paper suit, he asks me if I would 'like a cup of tea or coffee?' So civilised; why, yes I would! 'Tea, Earl Grey, Hot,' I replied in my best Jean Luc Picard. Cutriss then asked whether I wanted 'milk, honey or lemon,' and accepting that it may be a long while before I'd see such things again, I replied 'both honey and lemon'.

Later, at the station, an Officer gathered my clothing 'for forensics' and then stood me in a shower without soap; yes, without soap; very helpful indeed for those concerned I might have potent chemistry on my skin: not for a moment longer did they keep up that charade. (Forensics never actually did test my clothes or, strangely, anything directly on my lab bench).

After the doctor asked me a number of questions relating to mental health, I was booked on some cursory possession charges and escorted to a cell where I lay down in my fancy new prison blues: a jump suit type-thing. Then, in a moment of blistering clarity, I thought 'Wow, now I can rest'. So I closed my eyes and enjoyed the residual closed eye visuals of the last vestiges of my own acid: praise infinite ineffable *isness* for my life!

PPUK: *I think a lot of people's assumptions about being busted whilst high on acid would be that it might proliferate a 'freak out' of sorts. It appears for you, however, that it was a space in which to rest during the exteriority of Her Majesty's stress. Do you think there is something to be said for it being a meditative state, and is this skill to be cultivated?*

CH: Absolutely, realizing that I create, maintain and promote my mental weather provides me with both a profound privilege and responsibility to be here now, in the moment, without embellishment. Most of my suffering, when it occurs, comes from manifestations of my mind that may be illusory. If I'm suffering, what illusory reality did I create with my pattern recognition and creation system: what words did I say to myself? Have I created miscommunications, thwarted intentions, or unfulfilled expectations?

When Pike came up to me to arrest me, that was the current reality. I could either go with the flow or paddle upstream. I chose to go with the flow and the adventure of being arrested for making acid. I was joining the pantheon of incarcerated acid chemists: how cool was that? Later, in prison, away from most of the distractions of modern life, I realized how nice it was to have my own space to study, do yoga, dance, and be. When the door closed in the evening, it wasn't going to open again for at least 12-15 hours. In that cave, I found a contented silence within.

The experience was invaluable and rare. The message is perennial.

> **PPUK**: *When your case came to court you chose to defend yourself and use the arguments centred around cognitive liberty, therapeutic choice, and free religion. Unfortunately these arguments fell on deaf ears. After a number of unsuccessful appeals and an investigation into UK law and English Parliament, you came to understand the argument within the context of equal rights and equal protection. Could you elaborate on this shift please? And, moreover, what these positions could mean for today's court cases in Britain?*

CH: Well, trying to keep it brief, when I started the process I was arguing that the law itself was bad and that it must be struck down on the principles of cognitive liberty, therapeutic choice and freedom of religion: I would later see that these three principles can each be considered as facets of free thought. If we define thought deeply as cellular signalling pathways, each learned, or habituated, to over time - expressed genetically as 'instincts' or programs that run in the background 'unconsciously' - and we include what we neurotypically consider of as thoughts, those 'consciously' noticed semiotic snippets of information - signs, symbols, symptoms whizzing around our brains as mind manifestations - then we can span what any individual might conceive of as therapeutically efficacious for themselves, as that conception boils down to belief, some of which may get codified. Here, we run back into religion. They're one and the same: semiotic habituations.

Should we not be free to pursue whatever semiotic habituations we desire as long as we harm no others? After all, it is precisely what each of us have been doing since the dawn of life. Remember, folks, we have never died! We survived this long with the assistance of biochemical semiotic habituations. So it all boils down to freedom of thought, aka Cognitive Liberty. I want to play with my own mind as I see fit! But, I digress.

Eventually, after line by line study of the UK Misuse of Drugs Act 1971, with 'circles and arrows and paragraphs on the back', to paraphrase a friend, I began to see its regulatory mechanisms as ingeniously conceived by a genuine and caring Parliament, but it had a faulty master mechanism: *section 2(5)*, which regulates the Secretary of State's discretion in the promulgation and execution of the Act's regulatory structure. As stated, *s2(5)* gives arbitrary power to the Home Secretary to include a drug in the Act's controls. It was obvious to me that the Secretary, over time, had been biased toward familiar drugs like alcohol and tobacco and away from less or even unfamiliar drugs. So those who use these unfamiliar drugs suffer two arbitrary and unequal treatments, based on the familiarity to the majority of their drug of choice:

> *a failure to treat like cases alike,* viz *the unequal application of the Act to persons concerned with equally harmful drugs without a rational and objective basis; and*

> *a failure to treat unlike cases differently,* viz *the failure to regulate persons concerned in peaceful activities, re controlled drugs, differently from persons causing harm.*

Seeing the crux of the matter in this way allowed for a common law claim against the Home Secretary and the Advisory Council on the Misuse of Drugs for their administration of the Act. This leaves out the special pleadings on human rights grounds. Here it is simply the execution of a legislative discretion in an arbitrary manner. Theoretically, it is the duty of the court to check executive abuse of power in the administration of law.

If the Act were administered without the 'familiarity blind spot' and all drugs were included in the Act's control mechanisms, the Act itself, as written, is competent to make provisions for a fully regulated and lawful commerce in drugs. Each drug could have tailored regulations based on the best available science, in a manner that maximises benefits and minimises risks: this process could be led by the Advisory Council, as I believe the drafters of the law intended.

It's important to realise here that the Act is not about 'prohibition'. The Act has the inbuilt flexibility; remember, and the Act's regulatory mechanisms are, in my opinion, ingeniously conceived by a genuine and caring Parliament. We could, if the people were so minded, implement a version of Transform's Blueprint for Regulation right now, without need for any new primary legislation. All we need to do is establish and enact regulatory rules or secondary legislation.

Said another way, if the Home Secretary was so minded and Parliament didn't resist, then we could be buying *Cannabis* at the local drug store, chemist, pharmacy, in under three months. This under an Act of Parliament that I once thought was 'bad on its face'; nope, it's badly administered.

> **PPUK**: *This makes it sound like having cannabis in the shops is well within our grasp, but a lot of people still argue – especially many who wish to see proper legal, regulatory procedures in place - that it remains somewhat of a pipedream. For those who wish to see a change, especially along the lines you have just discussed, how do you think they might best proceed?*

CH: First, as I said about mental freedom above, it's about language. Stop talking about 'legalising' a substance. It's about property rights: possession, supply, production, export, import. These are actions by humans. That is the only thing a law can control. Drugs won't behave: they just are. Said another way: 'illegal drugs don't exist', only illegal actions.

The whole debate about slavery came down to the definitions and actions regarding property. If slaves were property and didn't own themselves then it was perfectly legal to be a slave owner. Once the concept got out that slaves were their own property, they could do with themselves as they saw fit, and possessing, supplying, producing slaves (often by rape) became a crime.

So when we talk of regulation, we mean regulating ourselves, our own actions. If I have a right to alter my mental functioning with drug A, why not drug B? On what rational basis can we distinguish the two. If, by consensus, we agree that a distinction exists then let's create a rational regulation that targets narrowly the action we seek to regulate. Second, spread a few memes: *Cognitive Liberty*, in particular. In 2006, the UK Home Secretary said:

> *A classification system that applies to [alcohol, tobacco and 'controlled drugs'] would be unacceptable to the vast majority of people who use, for example alcohol, responsibly and would conflict with deeply embedded historical tradition and tolerance of consumption of a number of substances that alter mental functioning*[1]

That's cognitive liberty for alcohol and tobacco users, so, why not extend the tolerance to my traditions, to my drugs of choice?

Finally, tell everyone that the Misuse of Drugs Act 1971 already has all the provisions in it to create a regulatory structure that provides for individual drugs of choice. See, *ss1, 2, 7(1)-(2), 22(a), 31(1)(a)* in particular. For instance, *Section 31(1)(a)* says:

> *(1) Regulations made by the Secretary of State under any provision of this Act –*
> *(a) may make* different *provision in relation to* different *controlled drugs,* different *classes of persons,* different *provisions of this Act or other* different *cases or circumstances;*

Is that enough 'differences' for you? The flexibility is enormous especially when combined with *s7*:

> *7. Authorisation of activities otherwise unlawful under foregoing provisions.*
>
> The Secretary of State may *by regulations – (a) except from section 3(1)(a) or (b), 4(1)(a) or (b) or 5(1) of this Act such controlled drugs as may be specified in the regulations; and (b)* make such other provision as he thinks fit for the purpose of making it lawful for persons to do things *which under any of the following provisions of this Act, that is to say sections 4(1), 5(1) and 6(1),* it would otherwise be unlawful for them to do.
>
> *Without prejudice to the generality of paragraph (b) of subsection (1) above, regulations under that subsection authorising the doing of any such thing as is mentioned in that paragraph may in particular provide for the doing of that thing to be lawful – (a) if it is done under and in accordance with the terms of a license or other authority issued by the Secretary of State and in compliance with any conditions attached thereto; or (b) if it is done in compliance with such conditions as may be prescribed* (Emphasis added)

The Secretary of State's power to prescribe, under *ss7(1)-(2)*, which of the offences, enumerated in *ss3-6*, apply to which controlled drugs makes plural 'regimes' possible. Add to this *s22*:

> *22. Further powers to make regulations.*
>
> *The Secretary of State* may *by regulations* make provision *– (a)* for excluding *in such cases as may be prescribed – (i) the application of* any provision of this Act which creates an offence; *(*Emphasis added*)*

Here, under *s22*, the Secretary to State can, by statutory instrument, exclude the application of *any* offence. This is an exceptionally wide power: if the Secretary was so inclined, and Parliament approved, personal possession of controlled drugs could be made lawful by the weekend. In short, educate yourself, speak accurately, speak often.

PPUK: *After being given an unbelievable 20 year sentence you were released earlier last year and deported from the UK. How have you enjoyed your new-found freedom, and have your views and resolve about entheogens changed?*

CH: As I said to Jon Hanna: 'Freedom is ace'. I stole that line from my exquisite English wife Charlotte. She and I took the opportunity to travel about 10,000 road miles through the Mountain and Pacific Western United States. We 'did' 11 states, 14 national parks, a dozen hot springs, many miles of wilderness hikes, made love by the light of the moon in the hot desert night, hunker down on the north rim of the Grand Canyon during a lightning storm, watched a full moon rise over a pink volcano as venus chased the sunset, hung on a bend of the Pit River making the fish dance by shadow casting, saw friends and family I had not seen in years, visited a few of the haunts of my youth, *ad infinitum*. Basically, we 'had' too many beautiful adventures to recount them all in this itty bitty space.

And then it happened, I now have new prisons: rent, a phone bill, insurance contracts, possessions to store and maintain, new needs and wants, and, gratefully, through the sweat of my brow, a lawful income to pay for them. I think prison is a state of mind: sure one cannot physically roam in a real bricks and mortar prison but my thoughts are subject to no rule outside or inside. And so today I find myself outside the 'ordinary' prison walls in 'the' Lavid Duke's E-Cat, that electronic dataerotrophic all-consuming surveillance prison of the United Corporate Nations (*read: 'The civilised world'*). Furthermore, I am now all too aware of the psychological shackles so many impose on themselves: somnambulating automatons wondering where they squandered their precious freedom away. So many hanging on in quiet desperation; and, not just the English as Floyd had it. Or as the modern Dread Pirate Roberts of Silk Road fame said:

Is it possible for someone locked in a cage to be freer than someone who isn't? What if they are free from limiting beliefs and can imagine experiences without limits, while the other limits themselves to a prison of dull routines?

More importantly for this tapestry: what the fuck is up with John Halpern patenting the word 'entheogen'? Now, thanks to him, we have 'entheogencorp.com'. Entheogen, a word laden with so much meaning for so many, has now been raped by commercial interest (alas, 'psychedelic. com' too is owned by a man with a Forbes profile). But I have come to believe, thanks to my ridiculously sensical wife, the neologistic experiment was won by Osmond. He nailed it with psychedelic. In my opinion, and I assume his, it is all mind-manifestations: 'we make shit up', that's what humans do!

But, let's not forget, I have written several articles from the perspective of 'an entheogenic chemist': a chemist that recognises my divine right to breathe air and love my fellow earthlings; a man who knows he is whole and complete, lacking no parts, though mindful improvements can be made. I have a deep affinity for the coining of the verbage *entheogenic* - that which recognises the power of mind, of theo-rising, of making shit up! So good at it, I am, that I believe the word goes a great distance to making our world; or more specifically, making my world. I program myself with my language. It's the same for law, for belief systems, for religions, and anyone who, like myself, is attached to the word and its entheogenic power.

So, yes, my view on entheogens has changed, I'm tired of people attributing anything 'god-like' or 'supernatural' to molecules. It's the affects/effects of our biochemistry attempting to make sense or wade through the molecular assault we have occassioned on ourselves. If we attribute meaning to it, that's our fault. I am responsible for the meaning I make; in re-cognising that, I can re-habituate my cognitions to more empowering interpretations.

PPUK: *Casey, thank you so much for taking the time to answer our questions. Blessings for your insight, and on all your future endeavours.*

CHAPTER 17

On the Nature of Psilocybe Folk
Psychedelic Psychoid Persons

by Jack Hunter

The very first time I consumed liberty cap mushrooms (*Psilocybe semi-lanceata*), I caught glimpse of an intangible, weirdly organic, world that overlay our own. As I looked into that strange place my perception was inundated with spiralling, earthy forms and twisting geometric motifs that faded in and out of my consciousness. The strangest thing I saw on that weird autumn night, however, was a procession of small, two-dimensional, goblin-like creatures in the grain of a wooden chest of drawers. They were dark and organic with long pointed noses and elfin ears. At the time I called them fairies. In the midst of the whirling, impersonal, fractal chaos these entities seemed to be moving along the grain with deliberate intent. The creatures regarded me with indifference when they noticed that I was staring, and continued on with their procession. Their apparent agency differentiated them from the seething psychedelic patterns that surrounded them, and suggested that they were something more than simple hallucinations. But if they were not simple hallucinations then what were they?

Encounters with apparently sentient entities while under the influence of psychoactive substances are well documented in the psychedelic literature. Terence McKenna, in *The Invisible Landscape*[1] (1975), described his encounters with weird insectoid entities during an ayahuasca trip in the Amazon jungle. Countless people have recorded their experiences of a distinctively feminine presence while smoking Salvia divinorum. Rick Strassman's 2001 book *DMT: The Spirit Molecule*[2] contains numerous references to meetings with insect-like and extraterrestrial beings during DMT trips under laboratory conditions. In his autobio-graphical book *Cosmic Trigger*[3], Robert Anton Wilson described an encounter with a dancing 'man with warty green skin and pointy ears' following a peyote trip, likening it to Carlos Castaneda's peyote encoun-ter with the spirit Mescalito, as described in *The Teachings of Don Juan*[4]. More recently parapsychologist David Luke has described numerous meetings with 'thousand eyed' sentient beings after smoking DMT[5]. Hun-dreds of other examples could easily be cited, but for the time being these cases will suffice in demonstrating that psychedelic entity encounters are far from uncommon.

Now, let us return to the question we began with: if these entities are not simple hallucinations then what are they? Robert Anton Wilson invoked Carl Jung's notion of the archetype in an effort to interpret his encounter with 'Greenskin.' Jungian archetypes are conceived as symbolically mean-ingful complexes emerging from the collective unconscious. It is tempting, when thinking about the unconscious, to conclude that anything that has its foundations in it must consequently possess no form of independent real-ity, but this is not necessarily the case. Jung's notion of the unconscious was far more expansive than we might at first imagine, he wrote 'a psycho-logical truth is... just as good and respectable a thing as a physical truth [because] no one knows what 'psyche' is, and one knows just as little how far into nature 'psyche' extends[6]'. I know Jung developed the concept of the 'psychoid,' which he considered to exist both inside the unconscious mind and outside in the objective world as a sort of transcendent entity. It could be that the entities encountered during psychedelic experiences par-take of a psychoid nature, requiring our perception and engagement to become tangible, and yet also possessing an external and independent nature of their own.

This notion accords well with the model of consciousness proposed by the early psychical researcher F.W.H. Myers, who held that conscious-ness consists of at least two streams, which he termed subliminal and supraliminal[7]. The supraliminal stream is the one we experience as our everyday consciousness and awareness, while the subliminal stream is usually imperceptible to our conscious experience. On certain occasions, however, aspects of the subliminal can cross the threshold and enter into our supraliminal consciousness, in the context of altered states of con-sciousness, for example. For Myers our conscious awareness operates somewhat like a lens focusing only on a narrow stream of our total con-sciousness, and so altered states of consciousness can, from Myers' per-spective, be thought of as movements of the lens to different aspects of consciousness. Like Jung's notion of the unconscious, Myers' subliminal mind was not restricted to the psyche of the individual but also included the possibility of external, independent, influences that are not always available to our experience, but that could be visible to consciousness if the lens of awareness was directed towards them. Could psilocybin mushrooms, and other psychedelic substances, provide a means for a refocusing of the lens of awareness, directing conscious experience towards subliminal psychoid entities?

It used to be taken for granted, as a working hypothesis, that the unusual experiences associated with the ingestion of psychedelic substances were a result of over-stimulation of the brain, resulting in sensory overload and heightened sensory experiences. The most recent neurophysiological research conducted on the effects of psilocybin (being the active psychedelic component present in magic mushrooms), on the brain, however, seem to challenge this assumption[8]. A recent study monitored the effects of psilocybin on the brain using fMRI scanning technology and revealed that, rather than promoting increased activity, psilocybin appears to reduce the blood-flow to certain areas of the brain. Psilocybin is not, therefore, exciting the brain, but is shutting down certain functions. Yet, despite this decrease in brain activity, conscious sensory experience is seemingly expanded. The potential implications of this are enormous, if speculative. This data could be taken as supportive of the notion that the brain is a kind of reducing valve for consciousness, analogous to Myers' lens of experience, which narrows our experience of consciousness. Consequently, when the activity of the brain is limited by the effects of psilocybin our conscious experience is expanded. This is very similar to Henri Bergson's notion of the brain as a filter for consciousness, filtering out aspects of consciousness that might otherwise get in the way of our basic survival needs. This idea was further expanded upon by the psychedelic pioneer Aldous Huxley who suggested, in his book *The Doors of Perception* (1954), that in order to make biological survival possible, 'Mind at Large has to be funneled through the reducing valve of the brain and nervous system.' What Bergson and Huxley are essentially suggesting is that in order to cope with the survival pressures that come with existing as three-dimensional physical entities, our consciousness needs to be focused on only a very narrow band of reality. If we were constantly aware of the whole of reality we wouldn't stand a chance as physical organisms trying to survive in a predatory physical world.

So, where does this get us in terms of thinking about the ontology of the 'fairies' I saw in my bemushroomed state, or of the various other entities encountered by human beings during the psychedelic experience? Not particularly far, unfortunately, though it does present us with a useful model, accompanied by some good evidence, that can accommodate such encounters. This should be seen as a springboard for further inquiry. We have a potentially workable model of consciousness that does not exclude the possibility of external influences, the next step is to attempt to verify whether or not these entities are indeed independent, or whether they represent aspects of our own consciousness made to appear independent. This is not going to be an easy task, though it is, I feel, an important one.

CHAPTER 18

Myco-Metaphysics
A Philosopher on Magic Mushrooms

by Peter Sjöstedt-H

This report and reflection of my, 'my', experience of magic mushrooms begins on a walk with my brother through paths and fields in an isolated Cornish landscape. It is late October and the weather is particularly foggy. We turn into a grazed set of fields facing north. I was later to discover that this set of conditions is considered the ideal for the occurrence of the most common, and amongst the most potent, magic mushroom on this planet: *Psilocybe semilanceata*, or, the *Liberty Cap*.

Fortunately my brother was an amateur mycologist, and so immediately recognised the distinctive appearance of these little fungi: a cream colouration throughout the thin, crooked stem and the bell-shaped cap. Most distinctive, though, was the 'nipple' apex. We spent a few hours gathering a hundred or so specimens. At home, I placed them to dry and began reading about the organism, chiefly to gauge the safety of its ingestion.

A few days later, on a Sunday afternoon now in London, I mix about fifty of the 'shrooms' into three pots of yoghurt, to avoid their earthy taste. My girlfriend is with me in our flat – it is important that she is in my company as a loving anchor to reality, 'reality', as my studies indicated that deep fear can arise in rare cases.

After an hour, not much has occurred. I feel somewhat light, but not much else. I read the newspaper, but lose interest. Half an hour later, I begin to feel disappointment because I am not experiencing the effects I had read others experience. But now a drunken state befalls me and I simply want it to end. If I had wanted to become drunk, I should have enjoyed the taste of a fine beer as well, rather than the muddiness of dried fungus.

As a result, I have a slight anxiety simply to return to my usual state of mind. But then I decide to consider this anxiety as a phase of the trip I realised was now, near two hours later, emerging. The anxiety left and the journey began.

I should say now that this new state of being consisted of a variety of quite different phases, both mentally and physically (if I may for now use that standard dichotomy). It was as if I had taken several distinct drugs one after the other, although certain features were constant such as spatial and temporal distortion. The first phase in fact began with spatial distortion. I looked at the printer whilst sitting at my desk – it seemed to expand slightly, then retract, as if (I think now) it had a ribcage and lungs within so to breathe. I then turned to the right and stared at a lit paper lampshade. Its two-tone yellow texture suddenly became three-dimensional, having a depth of a centimetre or so. Fantastical interwoven streams flowed thereon, resembling a choreographed serpent dance or an animated Celtic, Nordic and Saxon weave design, as witnessed on historic jewellery and weapons. It is speculated that the Vikings at least took another hallucinogenic, or entheogenic (enThorogenic), fungus – the fly agaric – which induced the berserker rage where the warrior became one with his wolf or bear shirt ('*ber-serk*').

Next, I stood up but noticed that I had lost some control of my body. My body weight now seemed to match that of a lunar walker; my mind, of a lunatic. I floated to the sofa, slumped down and closed my eyes. I was overcome by a rich, deep, warm, loving calmness. I felt more comfortable than I had ever felt in my thirty-odd years of life. An incident of the 'sublime' began on that sofa: I softly fell through a gigantic tunnel that had a diameter of miles, a tunnel filled with golden cloud somewhat reminiscent of candyfloss. Next to the tunnel was a similar but smaller tunnel that was somehow to the upper left of my vision. Certainly I experienced the sublime, but it was combined with a feeling of supreme warmth and bliss. I felt as if I were in a channel that transported beings between the different celestial cities found in a heaven. Here too, time distorted in the sense that I did not know whether I had immersed in this calm for a few minutes or a few hours.

The next step through the wardrobe revealed what seemed to be a portal to yet another reality. What I experienced with my eyes closed far exceeded what I experienced with those wide-pupiled eyes open: the most awe-inspiring patterns and space-scapes, perpetually in motion. I witnessed gigantic, multicoloured layers, now and again becoming more directly three-dimensional. It is difficult to describe, but sometimes a three-dimensional image became properly three-dimensional, such as the difference between seeing a three-dimensional object on television and seeing it in everyday reality. At that point, 'I' felt as if it were therefore 'real' (though I shall qualify that adjective and personal pronoun later).

In this inner world, where I felt as if I travelled through the universe, I at one point arrived at a superstructure of pointy luminescent sheets that converged at a centre point, like a star-sized, wide mechanical rose. This structure was a sentience, however; an alien being who tried to communicate with me. I here thought that perhaps (I was not certain) our search for alien life was restricted, as humanity was only looking for it in the eyes-open world, the world Immanuel Kant calls *phenomena*. Rather, we should realise that this other world I was accessing was the one that aliens used to make contact. Again, I was aware that I was speculating and certainly did not have the conviction of certainty that William James labelled *noetic* for mystical experiences. I did not know; I considered. But, as epistemology reveals, we cannot know, be certain of, much at all even in the phenomenal world. Even the great empiricist David Hume understood the problem of induction and causation which afflicts the science of men. A wishful thinker could have easily interpreted his experiences here as evidence of aliens, or even of God. The question concerned the veridicality (objective reality) of that which was experienced, and thus the fundamental nature of consciousness.

An early twentieth-century dominant school of thought, Logical Positivism (or Verificationism) would confer absolutely no veridicality upon such experiences. James' notion of noeticism would be shot down by the Positivists' 'Verification Principle', which claims that a statement can only be meaningful if it is either true by definition or if it can be verified by the senses. Alfred Jules Ayer was a notable and vociferous advocate of this school, explicitly applying it against any knowledge claims made by mystics. Many people still today harbour, unwittingly, this Verificationist ideology: if it cannot be proved, it cannot be true. However, Logical Positivism itself was forced to move on – due, ironically, to logical problems. When asked later in life, in the late 1970s, what the main shortcomings of the movement were, Ayer replied, 'Well ... nearly all of it is false!'[1]

Later still, a year before his death, Ayer had a near death experience. He wrote about it in an article in the *Sunday Telegraph* in 1988 entitled 'What I Saw When I Was Dead' – and though it was brought on by pneumonia, it might as well have been brought on by psilocybin. He wrote that whilst clinically dead, he

was confronted by a red light, exceedingly bright, and also very painful even when I turned away from it. I was aware that this light was responsible for the government of the universe. Among its ministers were two creatures who had been put in charge of space. These ministers periodically inspected space and had recently carried out such an inspection. They had, however, failed to do their work properly, with the result that space, like a badly fitting jigsaw puzzle, was slightly out of joint.

He later in the article remarkably remarked that,

On the face of it, these experiences, on the assumption that the last one was veridical, are rather strong evidence that death does not put an end to consciousness ... my recent experiences have slightly weakened my conviction that my genuine death, which is due fairly soon, will be the end of me, though I continue to hope that it will be. They have not weakened my conviction that there is no God.[2]

Interestingly, one of the main issues with Logical Positivism was the so-called 'Problem of Other Minds': how can I really know that other people, other beings, have minds? Of course, we assume that others have minds; but we cannot strictly prove it, we cannot verify it. We cannot, as it were, perceive the consciousness of another, despite perceiving their behaviour. Even with a brain scan, we can only infer (rather than experience) that a person has a mind – a very useful inference. Therefore, a statement such as 'He decided against it' would have to be meaningless for the Verificationists. Instead of abandoning belief in such everyday statements, most Positivists abandoned their creed.

However, this really led to the abandoning of one sinking ship for the embarking upon another fatefully leaking vessel: Behaviourism. If a statement such as 'You are satisfied' cannot be verified, some hardliners reasoned, then it must be because such statements do not refer to states of mind but merely to behaviour. Thus entered the prevalent Western academic notion that the mind, or consciousness, did not really exist. All statements about conscious states could be reduced to statements about behaviour. For instance, if someone said, 'I am happy', that happiness could ultimately be reduced to physical movements such as smiling, laughing, etc. There is no happiness, only behaviour. This seemingly incredulous ideology pleased many in the scientific field because, as the proverb goes, science would be happier if consciousness did not exist. Well, with this Logical Behaviourism, it did not exist. Neuroscience could steam ahead without being concerned with 'consciousness', now on a par with alchemy and alien abduction.

Apart from the ease it caused a lot of researchers, it also harmonised with a larger ideology that still prevails: Materialism: that each and every phenomenon can be essentially reduced to 'things' moving in space-time according to 'fixed laws'.

As the water started to flood into the Behaviourist vessel – mockingly reflected in the quip Behaviourist greeting, 'You're fine, how am I?' – a more serious crack manifested on the hull in the late 1990s: 'The Hard Problem of Consciousness'. This was really a centuries-old problem that had reasserted itself due to the implausibility of this Behaviourist modern paradigm and its materialist relations: Eliminativism, Functionalism, etc. The Hard Problem of Consciousness is that no matter the extent of knowledge concerning the brain and nervous system, one will never from that be able to sufficiently understand consciousness. 'Things' moving in space and time (viz. neuronal transmitters, ionic pulses, etc.), no matter the complexity, will never yield a knowledge of the consciousness which is, no doubt, correlated to that movement. Knowledge of movements cannot amount to knowledge of *qualia* (experience). As Frank Jackson once put it, in not so few words, a brain expert who has never experienced the qualia of redness will never gain a knowledge of redness through having a total knowledge of brain anatomy and function. Experience transcends neurology.

If I studied the activity of the brain of an octopus, two-thirds of which lie in its arms, I might gain an understanding of how certain physiological activities result in certain other physiological activities, such as neuronal pattern A relating to behaviour A. However, no matter how much I materially investigated, I would never actually know what it was like to be that octopus, to know how it experienced life. Logically speaking, it's not even necessary that eyes correspond to vision, or that ears correspond to sound. Even to human synaesthetes, these common correspondences do not attain; they can hear colours and see sounds. That the psilocybin of Liberty Caps is dephosphorylated to psilocin, which then mimics the effects of serotonin in the brain's serotonin receptors, etc., tells me little about the experiences correlated thereto. Even equipped with a total understanding of how psilocin acts upon the brain and body, one could not sufficiently know the experiences taking place because many such experiences are unknown, novel and because of this ineffable; and thus cannot be reported – and for mind-brain correlation, one needs that correlate: the mind report. Even if an octopus theoretically gave a report of its teuthological *qualia*, we humans would be none the wiser: there is even recent evidence that such cephalopods can 'see' with their skin[3]. Moreover, as I shall later mention, it may very well be the case that the brain does not completely produce the mind (that it does is an unproved assumption based on conflating correlation with causality). Knowledge is not reducible to moving matter.

This is to say, the Hard Problem of Consciousness can be seen as a disproof of Materialism.

With this in mind, one can be more open to the offerings of psychedelics. In fact, furthermore, psychedelic experience should be welcomed by researchers in the fields of philosophy of mind and neuroscience, as it once was in psychology, as it can present such awe-inspiring, unusual states of mind – an untapped ocean. To go beyond a mere physical understanding of the mind, to a thus metaphysical understanding, can be practically catalysed through these fungi. *Magic mycology is practical metaphysics.*

At one point a few hours into my magic myco tour, I noticed a cup of tea sitting in front of me as I lay on the sofa. I wanted it, but my desire found it very difficult to direct my body. Slowly I managed to move towards that hot drink, I crawled up to the table and demanded my body to at least sip the cup.

Whilst this overall tea motion was in play, a myriad of other thoughts, feelings and bizarre visions enveloped me. Most of these experiences were indescribable, I'm not even happy dividing the experience into that triad of words. If only the Behaviourists had tried such psychonautical substances, they might have realised the impossibility of their faith. How possibly could the behaviour that was the slow clumsy tea crawl executed by my body in any way translate into the psychedelic experiences I was having en route? In fact, for most of my voyage I was not behaving at all: I was lying still, eyes closed, traversing the universe, conversing with occult elves, insectoid aliens, deities–

God: I saw two flowing eyes staring at me. I considered them sentient and I still felt bliss. If I were already religious, I should probably have considered this to be proof of God. However, I realised that if I had not the cultural understanding of God from religion, I could not have interpreted my meeting as one with the Almighty. Secondly, as has been said of dreams, what really is the difference between dreaming that one met God, and actually meeting God in one's dream? There seems to be no experiential difference, either in dreams or during psychedelic experiences.

I could equally have interpreted this as a meeting with aliens desperate to make connections with human beings, or I could have interpreted it as a demon, or even as Satan. A spiritual experience must still be interpreted, and the tools used for interpretation are significantly cultural. The question though is whether religion emerged from such experiences in the past, or whether religion emerged from power structures, ancestor worship, anthropomorphism, linguistic twists, etc. I should argue that what we now call religion has a plurality of origins, drug-induced experiences being but one.

Writing of the devil, at one point I believed I was the devil, Satan himself. This was because, I think now, I saw many occult, demonic images but felt completely at ease; as if the dark spirits were my friends. One image I remember in particular was a sort of waterfall, shaped as a goat's head, from which fell and ran tens of wolves, goats and skulls towards me. It was in black and white, but covered simultaneously in multicolour. At another point, I saw a streaming wall of skulls and iron crosses. It was hell; but I liked it, I was at home here. So it dawned on me that I was probably the Prince of Darkness. I took this all very light-heartedly, despite the intensity of the images. Perhaps there was no real distinction between gods and devils – in Revelation 22:16 it states that I, Jesus, am Lucifer (Lucifer being the Latin for bringer of light, Venus). It was only post-biblical theologies that interpreted demons as the old pagan gods, Lucifer as the Devil, the fallen angel. As Nietzsche advocated, once we think in terms beyond good and evil (a dualism introduced by the Zoroastrians, advanced by the Christians), we will be able to interpret in a purer fashion. Dark demonic imagery is not necessarily 'evil'; a so-called 'bad' trip may only occur to those with deeply inculcated cultural value distinctions. If one is able to accept both creation and destruction as necessary elements of reality, one can accept life. In Jungian terms, to accept oneself involves accepting the Shadow archetype – a notion inspired by Nietzsche's strand of nihilism and Freud's similarly influenced 'Death Drive'.

Before I opened my eyes and entered the world of phenomena once more, another ostensible realisation dawned upon me: What was 'me'? I realised that what 'I' am/is, is only one 'thing' as a word. Really, 'I' is a conglomerate of many levels. Though I had come to this thought previously in life via the study of Kant, Nietzsche, and some psychology, I had never properly come to this feeling. At one level throughout the trip, I always considered reason to be there, as a judge, a viewer of what was happening to me. Though reason had lost his power over the body and was very easily sidetracked vis-à-vis 'his' line of thought. I considered reason as something that rolled on the underside of my skull, metaphorically. On another level was the unfolding of 'my' imagination. If this was merely imagination, it was also 'I' that was its author. But then on another level still 'I' – another 'I' – was watching this imagination unfold. Parts of the mind were watching other parts of the mind, so what part was 'me'? The Ancient Greek view that one watches a dream rather than has a dream would make this realisation less perplexing. Another level still of my self was my body. As I opened my eyes, I decided to try reading. Rather surprisingly, when I opened Nietzsche's *Thus Spoke Zarathustra*, the first sentence I encountered was, '"My ego is something that should be overcome": that is what this eye says.'

I was now moving a little more fluidly, normally. However, not all was as it seemed.

Not only was space being made a mockery of, but also time. As I waved my hand before me, it left a trail of itself. As I followed a lemniscate path with my hand, a lemniscate figure remained. The reason for this, it seemed to me, was that the present, the now, had extended its duration. What I saw and what I 'remembered' seeing were combined, giving the impression of a trail. The now had expanded to around five seconds – recent memory was perception, or rather perception and memory were not particularly distinct. It was not Schopenhauer's 'Eternal Now', but it was a longer now.

The great philosopher Henri Bergson's main ideas concerned time and perception, the mind and memory. Aldous Huxley employed Bergson's thought in his text, *The Doors of Perception* – probably the most celebrated psychedelic text in the athenaeum – wherein he describes and interprets his mescaline experiences in the 1950s, a time when such pharmaco-psychological adventures were seen in a more respectable academic light; before the prohibition imposed in the 1960s blacklisted this field of study, to the detriment of the advance of man.

For Bergson, all outer perception involves the contraction of memory: for example, the colour red is partly a collection, a contraction, of billions of certain electromagnetic waves. Without 'memorising' the initial waves, the latter would not engender the redness. It seemed as if this automatic human memory-for-perception function had allowed more of the past into the contraction with regard to my lemniscate trail. Other life forms may very well have other durations of memory for perception, thus perceiving the universe very differently from we humans. This would entail perceiving time at relatively different speeds, a notion recently acknowledged in the scientific literature[4]. The magic mushroom, in other words, grants one entry to non-human modes of time and sensation. And it is worth noting that there is no absolute, correct, real 'speed of time'. Nietzsche, when explaining the philosophy of flux as advocated by Heraclitus, illustrates strikingly this time/speed variability:

The inner life of various animal species (including humans) proceeds through the same astronomical time-space at different rates ... [Reduce] sensation threshold by one-thousandth ... then every four hours we would watch winter melt away, the earth thaw out, grass and flowers spring up, trees come into full bloom and bear fruit, and then all vegetation wilt once more ... a mushroom would suddenly sprout up like a fountain. [Decelerate more] the solar ecliptic would appear as a luminous bow across the sky, as a glowing coal, when swung in a circle, appears to form a circle of fire ... Whatever remains, the unmoving, proves to be a complete illusion, the result of our human intellect ... forms exist only at certain levels of perception.[5]

Bergson argued that the brain did not produce the mind, but merely channelled it according to human practical requirements – a theory that would still entail mind-brain correlation in scans. The brain would hence be a necessary but not sufficient cause of standard *homo sapien* consciousness. Therefore, mind would be antecedent to brain, and far overreaches the limited versions of consciousness that are useful to our survival and development. It is the practical will that determines the extent of human consciousness – thus if one theoretically closed the will, one could thereby open the doors to that greater overarching mind. Applying Bergson's dense theory[6], one can say that psychedelics act as will inhibitors, they breakdown the normal functioning of the brain, so that consciousness is not restrained in this way. In other words, psychedelic compounds do not only produce 'hallucinations' (everyday reality also being a hallucination, in the strict sense), but they also allow access to a reality usually denied. It would not be in our interest to be constantly awestruck by sublime celestial cloud tunnels and so on. In this light, psychedelics can be seen as a temporary death; as such Ayer's near-/death experience, above, resembling a psychedelic experience, is made sense of.

Furthermore, in Bergson's thought there is no actual distinction between the subject ('me') and the object ('it') because a perception exists in both, as a perception is one process that is ultimately indivisible, even at the bodily limit. A perception of a star is both part of that star and part of you, the process of its light entering and adjusting your body is one process; the consciousness lies throughout, not merely within the brain. However, it is in our biological interest to dissect reality into parts so that it can be manipulated through reason: medicine and weapons lying at either end of this practical spectrum. But these useful abstract distinctions (words such as 'me', 'star', 'perception') can be annulled through psychedelic intake, thus providing an intuition of unity, empathy, identity, etc – a common henological insight experienced not only in the psychedelic state but also in mystical states. In fact, the study of 'henology' (the metaphysics of radical transcendence to The One) is rather old and has been attributed notably to the neo-Platonist Plotinus, of the third century AD, who inspired much of the mysticism in subsequent religious thought.

But the ultimate unity of all does not contradict the overall multiplicity of power structures. An organism must exploit its environment to live: it must digest external organisms, re-constitute the atmosphere through its breathing, and so on. The psychedelic experience can provide one with intuitions of both aspects of reality – there is no moral hierarchy in total acceptance. The transcendent One must interweave with the immanent Nietzschean Wills to Power.

At a later point, I started writing notes, quite odd as I look at them now, in order not to forget my trip. I noted that art and logic were essentially the same thing, in that they put 'things together, under a scheme (composition in art, taxonomy in biology)'. This seemed somewhat profound at the time, but now seems a little shallow. However, I do believe that this idea and others could be investigated further, and therefore realise that the fungus liberated my thoughts enabling seeds to be sown for development when the mind is less free but more focused. The term 'Liberty Cap' is hence quite fitting for such mushrooms – fungi for Philosophy.

CHAPTER 19

Seismographic Psychedelia
Reflections on the Direct Influence of Psychedelics on Art

by Henrik Dahl

> *Generally, one might argue, writers and musicians are*
> *more associated with psychedelics than are visual artists*
> – Robert C. Morgan

Psychedelics often trigger a rich flood of visual content. For instance, one may experience highly intricate patterns, otherworldly landscapes and mysterious beings - some angelic, others demonic. Colours are frequently perceived as being extremely intense and objects may transform into bizarre and unthinkable shapes. Surely visions like these must be of great interest to visual artists. Still, most psychedelic culture researchers will find it hard to come up with a satisfying list of visual artists who acknowledge the importance of psychedelics in their work. Why is this the case? When it comes to writers and musicians, examples are plenty. Shouldn't there be as many, if not more, visual artists associated with psychedelics?

Admittedly, there is a lot of psychedelic art out there. Usually though the term is used to describe a particular aesthetic rather than art directly influenced by psychedelic drugs. Surprisingly little has been written about art that is psychedelic in the true sense of the word. The typical take on the subject is exemplified by art critic Ken Johnson who is the author of *Are You Experienced? How Psychedelic Consciousness Transformed Modern Art*: 'While I think it would be a worthy project for a sociologist or historian to find out who did what, when, and where, to provide some empirical grounding for speculations about the influence of drugs on art, I am neither equipped for nor inclined to do that job. What interested me was not necessarily the influence of drugs on particular individuals but the influence of psychedelic culture in general on artists[1]'. A similar approach is found in David S. Rubin's *Psychedelic: Optical and Visionary Art Since the 1960s*, which explores the visual impact that psychedelic culture has had on artists working over the past five decades.

Although Johnson and Rubin have done a great and much welcome job with their respective books, they raise an important question: How many of the artists described as 'psychedelic' actually feel comfortable with being categorised in such a way? In today's highly professionalised art world it's likely that at least *some* artists find the association problematic. Reasons for this may vary of course, but the connection to drug culture is probably one of them. Perhaps this is why Johnson points out that readers of his book are advised 'not to assume that any artist discussed... has even used drugs at all or would agree that drug-induced experience has affected their art[2]'.

Obviously, to be certain that a psychedelic has influenced an artwork one needs some sort of testimony from the artist that confirms the association. This fact dramatically narrows the number of artworks that are clearly induced by a psychedelic. With that said, many artists have openly ascribed psychedelic experiences as a major influence on one or several of their artworks.

Discussions about psychedelic art are often reduced to speculations, where critics sometimes see 'trippy' influences in artworks that in reality have little to do with the psychedelic experience, mistaking it for themes such as dreams states, New Age spirituality or the occult. This essay is a modest attempt at approaching the subject differently; rather than looking at art influenced by psychedelic culture as a whole, I will present some of the art that has been *directly* influenced by psychedelics.

A key figure when it comes to western art directly influenced by psychedelics is the Belgian-born French visual artist and writer Henri Michaux. Already in the 1960s he was looked upon as 'a pioneer in psychedelic art[3]'. His perhaps most notable work is *Miserable Miracle*, containing both his writings and drawings, published for the first time in French in 1956. The book was the result of the author's experiments with mescaline. In his dissertation *A History of Irritated Material: Psychedelic Concepts in Neo-Avant-Garde Art*, Danish art historian Lars Bang Larsen calls Michaux's drawings 'seismographic', describing them as 'pulsating, *brut* landscapes[4]'.

Michaux wasn't the only westerner experimenting with psychedelics at the time. Two years before *Miserable Miracle* came out, Aldous Huxley described his experiences on mescaline in his essay *The Doors of Perception*. Still, *Miserable Miracle* is an important work. Not least because of the inclusion of Michaux's psychedelic artworks. Incidentally, the same year as *Miserable Miracle* was first published, psychiatrist Humphry Osmond coined the word 'psychedelic' in a correspondence with Huxley. However, since Michaux was making his drug experiments long before 'psychedelic' became a catch phrase in the sixties counterculture, Larsen aptly describes Michaux as a 'proto-psychedelic artist[5]'.

Henri Michaux continued his explorations with mescaline, resulting in additional books on the subject. In 1963, he also made an educational film called *Images du monde visionnaire* for Swiss pharmaceutical company Sandoz (recognised by psychedelicists as the company where Albert Hofmann worked when he first synthesised LSD in 1938.) Michaux's film was made in collaboration with French filmmaker Eric Duvivier for the purpose of demonstrating the hallucinogenic effects of mescaline and hashish. Given the limitations of the technology at the time, the film's psychedelic effects looks a bit bleak and feel rather unconvincing today and, according to an article on book publisher Strange Attractor's website, Michaux himself was said to have been quite disappointed by the result. One may wonder if this is a common reaction among artists trying to depict psychedelic experiences. If that is the case, it's possible that many artists avoid such attempts.

Although Michaux's drawings were induced by a psychedelic drug, it wasn't until the mid to late sixties that psychedelic art became recognised as a distinct artistic expression of its own. An early proponent of the style during this era was American painter Isaac Abrams. In 1965, he had his first LSD session with psychologist Stanley Krippner. According to the blog Transpersonal Spirit, the experience gave him a vision of what he felt psychedelic art would look like. Abrams' artworks display oceanic, cosmic and microscopic motifs, exemplified by his 1968 painting *Cosmoerotica*. Still actively pursuing his art, he has stayed true to the artistic style he envisioned on his first acid trip.

As a result of the popularisation of LSD in the sixties, many visual artists experimented with the drug. It's easy to assume that those artists were automatically incorporating their experiences in their art. However, that was not always the case. German-born painter Mati Klarwein, known for painting the cover of Miles Davis' classic jazz album *Bitches Brew*, says his experiences with psychedelics never inspired his art in any major way. Instead, according to his biography on Matiklarwein.com, his inspiration came from extensive travelling and the artist's interest in non-western deities and symbolism.

One who ascribed great importance to psychedelics though was Swedish poster artist Sture Johannesson. In his piece *Psychedelic Manifesto* published in the Swedish magazine Ord & Bild, phrased in his typically humorous and anarchistic style, the artist immodestly promotes psychedelics saying, 'The cultural worker's most important task in the future is to spread information about these matters. Psychedelic drugs mean freedom, equality and brotherhood[6]'.

Between 1967 and 1969, Johannesson made a series of posters called *The Danish Collection*. They have stood the test of time surprisingly well and, apart from becoming collector's items, they are regularly exhibited at museums around the world. Included in the series is *Andrée Will Take A Trip* (1969). The poster, arguably one of his most complex and captivating works, shows a series of small photographs taken during Swedish engineer S.A. Andrée's balloon expedition to the North Pole in 1897, a misadventure that ended in the death of Andrée and his group. The photos are arranged against a pink background and at the top of these is a quote associated with William S. Burroughs saying, 'Anything which can be done chemically can be done by other means!' Lastly, much like a hallucination, three huge but delicately designed yellow letters placed in the centre of the image spells out the word 'LSD'.

An artistic genre that is often associated with the use of psychedelics is Visionary Art. Artists working in this style often depict visions experienced while in altered states. Although far from being the only source of inspiration, many visionary artists acknowledge the importance of psychedelics in their artistic process. The genre's association with mind-expanding drugs is evident in *First Draft of Manifesto of Visionary Art* written by visionary artist Laurence Caruana, where he discusses psychedelics at length. Interestingly, this type of art may have a particular function for those who view it: 'It is no secret that many Visionary works of art are designed to be viewed 'with the aid of mind-altering substances", he wrote in the manifesto[7].

One of the foremost artists working in the visionary style is Alex Grey. A prolific painter, his artworks have appeared on several album covers and his 1990 art book *Sacred Mirrors: The Visionary Art of Alex Grey* has been translated into several languages and is still in print. In the mid-seventies, while on LSD with his future wife, the artist Allyson Grey, Alex experienced what would prove to be a pivotal moment in his career as an artist. In a 2008 interview with SFGate.com, Alex said the trip made him interested in the study of consciousness, and that he started making drawings of what he had seen. For Allyson the experience turned out to be equally profound, saying it 'was to become the subject of our art for a lifetime' (Allysongrey.com). Alex's *Universal Mind Lattice* (1981) and Allyson's *Jewel Net of Indra* (1988) are both depictions of their LSD trip.

Another visionary artist associated with psychedelics is the Peruvian painter Pablo Amaringo. Amaringo, a *vegetalista* who depicted visions on ayahuasca, was brought to attention by ethnopharmacologist Dennis McKenna and anthropologist Luis Eduardo Luna. At Luna's suggestion Amaringo started painting his ayahuasca visions, which resulted in the co-authored book *Ayahuasca Visions: The Religious Iconography of a Peruvian Shaman* published in 1999. Apart from being a painter, Amaringo was the art teacher at his Usko-Ayar School of Painting and was supervising ayahuasca retreats.

Most visionary artists are highly skilled at their craft. According to Laurence Caruana, 'as precise a rendering as possible is absolutely necessary for vision-inducing works. Fine lines, gradual transitions, infinite details - there is no limit to the pains endured nor the patience required to successfully render a vision into image form[8]'. One may wonder at what length the complex nature of altered states of consciousness – including those triggered by psychedelics – has affected the technical abilities of artists working in the visionary style. It's possible that the sometimes incredibly detailed visions seen on mind-expanding drugs have forced these artists to perfect their work considerably more than had they worked in another artistic field.

When discussing artists who use psychedelics one should keep in mind that very few of them are likely to be making art while actually under the influence. For example, in an interview published on Historygraphicdesign.com in 2002 San Francisco poster artist Victor Moscoso strongly opposes to the idea: 'People ask me, 'Did you draw on acid?' Draw on acid? That's like drawing while you're tumbling down a flight of stairs. Are you kidding? With you dying and being re-born, having an understanding of the molecular structure of your body and of the cosmos at the same time. Drawing is absurd. You can't do it! Whatever you draw will not come close to what you can see, or perceive.'

Most artists using psychedelics would probably agree with Moscoso. Yet there are several examples of artists who have made art while they were on mind-expanding drugs. In 1990, Charles Ray shot a self-portrait when he was under the influence of LSD, resulting in his artwork *Yes*. Another contemporary artist making art while on LSD is Rodney Graham, whose film *The Phonokinetoscope* is a 2001 re-enactment of Albert Hofmann's legendary LSD bicycle trip in 1943. Also in 2001, Bryan Lewis Saunders made a series of self-portraits while on a variety of drugs, including psilocybin mushrooms and DMT. The three artworks mentioned pose the question of how these artists actually managed to make art while tripping. In all likelihood, they either made their artworks while they were coming down from their trips, or their doses were low from the beginning. In the case of Graham, he is quoted on Ubuweb.com saying he ingested 'a blotter'. Considering the fairly low doses usually distributed on blotter acid, Graham's trip was likely rather mild compared with Hofmann's, making the former's re-enactment a less dramatic event.

Why are relatively few artists associated with psychedelics? I can think of several possible eximagine.

CHAPTER 20

Cultivating the Teacher

Parallels in Sufism and the use of Psilocybin Mushrooms as a Spiritual Tool

by James W. Jesso

Sufism can be loosely described as the mystical school of Islam. I personally know little of this way of life as it is expressed in dedicated seekers, I am merely one who is interested in some of the founding principles it presents. In that interest, and in reading a book called *The Knowing Heart* by Kabir Helminski, I have begun to explore the applicability of certain Sufi principles as they relate to using psilocybin (magic) mushrooms as a tool for psychospiritual maturation. Specifically, this essay will explore the correlations related to the Sufi principles of *Dervish* and *Shaikh* (the relationship between student and teacher) and the role of *spiritual community*.

The intention here is not to promote Sufism but to elucidate how one can apply some of its principles in their relationship to mushrooms (or any visionary medicine) to create a student/teacher exchange between oneself and the visionary experience mushrooms occasion. If there are principles in a tradition, society, philosophy, religion, etc. that are found to widely apply outside of their cultural context, this offers support in the validity of those principles being cross-cultural in some sense. Thus also open to the public domain of human life without need for cultural appropriation. Sufism, as a way of life that is said to engender an increasing expression of spiritual maturity in the dedicated participant, seems to offer this caliber of applicable principles. In particular, some of these principles flow beautifully with the use of psilocybin mushrooms as a tool for cultivating spiritual maturity as well. In exploring the relationship between these Sufi principles and the use of psilocybin mushrooms as a tool for personal development, I hope to recapitulate these principles from their religious context for applicability and use within a personalized mushroom practice.

Before we continue with this essay, it is important to address the point that I will be frequently referring to new or loaded terms. I will do my best to define these terms as the text moves along to ensure the reader is able to understand what my intended use of them is. One of these terms is 'God'. I have often defined my use of 'God' simply as a term to reference the *All That Is, All At Once*. In *The Knowing Heart*[1], Helminski offers this description of Sufism's philosophical take on God, (it can be applied throughout the rest of this essay as the intention behind my use of the word as well):

> *Reality, the Source of Life, the Most Subtle State of Everything. The love of God is the love of the greatest Truth. This question concerns Reality, not religion. The 'love of God' is our essential relationship with what is most real*[2].

I touched on the relationship between Sufi principles and psilocybin mushrooms in my book *Decomposing The Shadow*. In the section titled 'God and Surrender', I write briefly on the correlations between accessing 'awareness of God' in Sufism and the process of *surrender* within a psilocybin experience:

> [It] *is stated* [*in Sufism that*] *those who love God are gifted three blessings: Islam (submission/surrender), Iman (faith) and Ihsan (awareness of God). Mushrooms can open our psychoemotional perception with such force that we may have no other choice but to give into its power (Islam) and have faith or trust in our self (Iman) that we will come through it alive. It is in this surrender and trust that we may get a glimpse of the true depth of spirit (Ihsan)*[3].

Since writing on this subject, I have further explored Sufism to find several other correlations between it and accessing, navigating and integrating the spiritual psychedelic experience. Such as the premise of a divine creative principle manifesting in all reality, encompassed in the Qur'an quote 'Wheresoever you look is the face of God' (2:115), and there being a capacity within the human being for perceiving an imaginal inner-world, full of symbolic meaningfulness rendered as visions and engaged through the active imagination. I have also found several of the principles for integrating spiritual perception into daily life and the path of Sufism in general to be in accordance with my personal practice with psilocybin mushrooms. Could the relationship between various principles in Sufism as a way to God and practice with visionary medicines such as psilocybin mushrooms, as a way to God, be representative of these principles as being a diversely applicable means to psychospiritual maturity[4]? Maybe, but for the purpose of this essay we will keep the inquiry into exploring the application of some of these principles in psilocybin experiences.

In *Decomposing The Shadow*, I offer a framework for psilocybin mushrooms as being a tool for catalysing increased emotional potency and self-awareness. In supporting the emergence of both the light and dark elements of the psyche, the cathartic release of repressed emotions, and exposure to a grander expression of self, the mushrooms can work as a teacher or a guide in one's process of psychospiritual maturation. I offer how to better occasion such types of experiences, how to navigate them and the psychological, emotional and spiritual mechanisms associated. I speak of offering oneself in respect to the mushroom as one's teacher and also the awareness that it is not the mushrooms but the *self* awakened in relationship the mushroom, that offers this guidance. The Sufi principles of *dervish*, *shaikh* and *spiritual community* helps to expand on how to better access and apply this teacher/guide relationship.

A *dervish* is a person who has committed themselves completely to 'the love of God' (ultimate truth) above all things through apprenticeship to their *shaikh*. A *shaikh* is also a *dervish*, though one who has committed themselves long enough to reach a point of becoming a teacher, one who is spiritually mature. The shaikh is not considered to be a being to worship, such as a living god, but as a being of inspiration and guidance towards maturity within a spiritual community. A spiritual community is group of dedicated participants whose intention is deepening their relationship to God.

'The shaikh does not gather power or privilege for himself or herself but is the servant of the yearning of the dervish's heart[5]'. This is to say that the shaikh is a teacher who has dedicated himself or herself as a dervish to God through offering themselves as a servant to the yearning of their student's process of maturity, and in their relationship to God. This is cultivated through *Rabita*, a connection of love. In many ways, this is essentially a relationship of offering and receiving love and respect through student and teacher as a means to deepen 'love of god' and integrate spiritual wisdom.

In Sufism, according to Helminski, it is understood that 'the truth is a 'trackless land' [and] one attains wisdom primarily through one's own experience, independent of guidance[6]'. Yet, it is also understood that the unconscious guidance offered by the immature human environment of conventional society, played out through the ego, is not one what will ultimately lead to spiritual maturity. In this understanding, it becomes highly functional to create a spiritual community that has a spiritually mature person or persons as example to aspire to and be inspired by. Else wise, one may simply cycle the same patterns of egotism almost indefinitely. In

Sufism, this is someone (the shaikh) who has come to fully embody *baraka* (grace) and *Rabita* in their relationship to God.

In Islam every human being has a direct relationship to the divine. In Sufism, however, this individual's relationship with the Divine is assisted by a sharing of mind with someone who has broken through the barrier that separates the alienated self [(ego)] from the wholeness of mind, which is transpersonal[7].

The dynamics of the relationship between student and teacher in this tradition work as a feedback loop. The shaikh is a servant of the dervish's yearning heart. Yet, the shaikh's ability to offer themselves in a way that allows for the dervish's advancement is dependent on how the dervish engages the shaikh. Essentially, a great teacher is the result of a great student and vice versa. Ideally, within the spiritual community, the students create a bond together that mutually empowers the students, and the teacher, through recognizing each other for their gifts and growth, holding each other accountable for their actions. All of this would be founded around ethical behavior, love, grace, respect, trust, and dedication, creating a field of support towards spiritual maturity for all parties[8].

Furthermore, it is also understood around some traditions of Sufism that the shaikh is merely an expression of the student's inner wisdom. This is why it is said that a great shaikh is the result of a great student. When a student offers the perception of reverence and wisdom in the teacher, those characteristics are reflected back to the student. The wisdom of the teacher is an objectified reflection of the student's inner-wisdom being played out through a relationship of Rabita. This is also why it is important to have the teacher as one who is spiritually mature, as spiritual maturity is an expression of 'someone who has broken through the barrier that separates the alienated self [ego] from the wholeness of mind[9]'. They have been able to release the assumptions and projections readily played out by the ego so as to work as clear mirrors for the wisdom shining out through the student's humble dedication.

We can see an example of how the shaikh is an expression of the dervish's inner wisdom in the great Sufi poet Rumi's relationship to his shaikh, Shams Tabrizi. After Shams disappeared, Rumi spent much time mourning his loss, searching for him. Eventually Rumi realized that to seek for Shams was unnecessary because all that he sought from his teacher was available within himself.

Why should I seek? I am the same as
He. His essence speaks through me.
I have been looking for myself!
  -Rumi[10]

It is here that we will begin to explore how this relates to psilocybin mushrooms. As mentioned earlier, I consider the use of psilocybin as a potential tool towards similar results as mentioned in Sufism, spiritual maturity. The mushroom can work as a guide in this process. But how does one obtain this guidance and who/what is guiding us? The mushroom?[11] And, how does this relate to Sufism?

Sufism speaks of the shaikh as one who has 'broken through the barrier that separates the alienated self from the wholeness of mind, which is transpersonal[12]'. This is exactly what the mushroom chemically unlocks for us. When one takes psilocybin mushrooms, the neurological actions being facilitated include decreased blood flow (and thus functioning) to the very areas of the human brain associated to maintaining ego self-identity patterns and the structured flow of information, especially the medial prefrontal cortex and the posterior cingulate[13]. In creating this neurological change, one of the associated experiential effects of psilocybin can be described as connecting to a world of transpersonal self-identity. Thus, the mushroom may very well biochemically activate oneself into a state of mind similar to that proclaimed of the shaikh.

There is a problem that arises here, however, as the potential results of a psilocybin experience are highly mutable and dependent on set (as in mindset or how we perceive the substance and occasioned experience), setting (as in the physical environment), dosage (how much of it we take) and how we integrate the experience. Just because the state of mind occasioned by psilocybin has the potential to employ shaikh-like awareness, does not mean that one's use of them makes one an awakened being. It is highly dependent on the aforementioned elements as to whether or not that awakening will occur within the participant. And furthermore, it must be understood that even if it does occur, the biochemical change it is sourced in will eventually wear off and the ego (alienated self) identity will return. However, it is possible to occasion experiences that awaken this type of awareness and engage them in a way that brings the lessons offered within those experiences back into the normal ego life. Over time, this may help us achieve fuller expressions of psychospiritual maturity.

Decomposing The Shadow outlines a complete cognitive model for the type of experiences that can potentiate these results. Expanding on what is presented there, it is possible to engage shaikh-like awareness with the mushroom experience but, as mentioned, it is all dependent on how one engages it.

Respect is the foundation of any constructive relationship; be it with a practice, person, or medicine. We are entering an exchange with an organism from which we are hoping to garner insight and/or healing. It is important to treat it with respect as we will gain more from the experience in this way. Respect is one of the manners through which we increase our receptivity to the mushroom's lessons about self *and life as a whole.*[...]

The source of an experience with psilocybin is not the mushroom itself, it is only the catalyst. The source of the experience is within us. So when we show respect to the experience and the substance that occasioned that experience, we are actually showing respect to an aspect of self. *This respect for* self *is a key element in utilizing psilocybin for personal growth*[14].

Helminski says that in Sufism a great shaikh is still an apprentice to something grander than itself. He also says what defines a shaikh as 'great' is how they are engaged by their students. It is the student who holds the shaikh in the reverence of being a 'great shaikh' that allows both to obtain the benefits of such an exchange. I present the same perspective here. If one offers reverence to the awakened-self occasioned by mushrooms as being a source of spiritual guidance and wisdom, one can obtain the benefits of such an exchange. Yet in order to do this, we must be able to hold trust for ourselves and the potential of what this experience offers as well as the *languages* we have to understand it, which takes time and commitment to develop.

We can help this process along by becoming students, not of the mushroom, but of the awakened-self. If we choose to build Rabita, a connection of love, founded on respect and reverence to that expressed element of self, we can build that self inside of us. At first, the mushroom-awakened self is highly limited in its scope as we, the student, are unfamiliar with its teachings. We are not yet familiar with how to be a student of this self, nor have we engaged the experience in a way that offers opportunity for the mushroom awakened-self to even be a dervish. In the early stages of this relationship, the calibre of wisdom that emerges is usually too novel or odd to be properly applicable in daily life; we lack the conceptual framework to navigate the experiential wisdom of the awakened-self in a functional way[15]. Yet in time, if we choose to engage the mushroom experience as students of the awakened-self, of our *self*, we cultivate a relationship to our inner wisdom. We do this by exploring the mushroom awareness with a systematic approach founded on this student/teacher perspective and in time build a sense of trust in ourselves, in that what the mushroom exposes us to (a deeper expression of our emotional connection to God, the essential transpersonal reality), as well as a conceptual framework to functionally navigate and apply it in daily life.

Relating this to Sufism, we choose to awaken the dervish (seeking apprentice) in the mushroom awakened shaikh (one who has embodied the wholeness of mind) and allow that expression of our self to explore and learn. We do this by becoming a student who honors and reveres the inner shaikh to a point where, in time, that shaikh, awakened in its exploration, has a wisdom that is accessible to the now familiar student (ourselves).

This established relationship of trust enables us to not only visit the awakened-self, but also integrate its wisdom into one's self-identity as we learn to apply it in our daily lives. Learning the applicability of wisdom offered in explorations with the mushroom comes through familiarizing ourselves with the dynamics of the experience, through learning how to engage ourselves and the world around in a manner that will offer personal benefit. Doing so can be benefited by 'spiritual community' or a group of people exchanging with each other on the foundation of ethical behavior, love, grace, respect, trust. Yet, it may also hinder us from true wisdom.

The process of properly integrating the wisdom of transpersonal self-identify can be benefited by connecting with others who are able to help us feel acknowledged in our growth and hold us accountable for our changes. I believe this is what Terence McKenna meant when he said 'find the others'; find those who have become students of the awakened-self so as to better help each other achieve fuller integration of the wisdom it offers[16]. This doesn't necessarily mean that one finds a group to talk about their experiences directly, but to simply share in communion with good people who have had similar experiences of awakening. Often, we speak to explain our psychedelic experiences too soon and miss the grander wisdom offered by constraining it into the only language the ego has available to explain it with at the time. It is best to wait. In a Sufi spiritual community, one doesn't speak of their religious experiences with each other, only with the shaikh. And the same may apply to psychedelic experiences as well. It is often best to communicate an expression of what has been learned in action and composure, more than in retelling the story. But of course, this is dependent on the context and the point of understanding one may be regarding their experiences. Eventually, the sharing of stories may be the very thing that supports others in their development towards maturity. This is a rather grey zone and there are no rules to define when or what works best to share one's stories.

This essay clearly does not intend to say that Sufism promotes, requires or is based on the use of mushrooms. It offers an outline to how Sufi principles can apply outside of their specific religious context. Like in Sufism, one can cultivate spiritual maturity and be empowered in their life and potential wisdom by becoming an honest student (dervish) of their transpersonal identity (shaikh) through a relationship of love and dedication their inner-wisdom accessed by psilocybin mushrooms.

However, and somewhat paradoxical to this entire essay, with any and all belief systems, whether they be attached to a religious text or a psychedelic experience, there are no guarantees that any of it will get you closer to spiritual maturity or God in any way. Sometimes these belief systems may help in navigating our experiences of life beyond the established ego and in turn cultivate a relative sense of God through directing the way we live. But they will inevitably hurt our development if they are not released in favor of simply being ourselves without imposed expectations.

In regards to the Sufi path of the 'seeker' and 'spiritual maturity' in general: Does creating an identity founded on being in search of something ever bring a sense of having found that which we seek? Who determines who as spiritually mature? Who determines the premise of cultivating spiritual maturity as all that important anyways? Is it someone outside of ourselves? Is this destination of maturity the point to life? If not, then is the *point* the journey? If the point is the journey, is there really any need to seek anything? Have we not already arrived exactly where we need to be? Of course, the premise of exploration and personal transformation holds a potential value to the individual and the development of what is described as spiritual maturity can offer positive effects in ones quality of life. In that way, both the use of psilocybin mushrooms and Sufism may offer the framework to encourage this. But again, who determines how and who we are suppose to be in life and what direction our journey should go?

Personally, with this question in mind, I rest with more confidence on the direct experience of psilocybin than the externalized direction of a religious belief system. A psilocybin experience does not require a belief system, nor, as outlined here, does it need anyone else to inform you of how, what or who you are supposed to be according to an externalized value system. It opens the option to journey through new perspectives on ourselves and in that way, maybe counter to what I offered here, the psilocybin experience isn't so much about spiritual maturity as it is about potentiating novelty in the journey we are already on. Of course, as stated earlier, having a systematic approach or framework for psilocybin experiences can help us to integrate those direct experiences, that is what this essay is all about. But the frameworks only have as much value as they are personally functional, the rest can be tossed in favor of what works best for the individual.

I ultimately feel that only through learning how to be love in and for yourself in the present moment, seeing the magic in the ordinary, without any belief systems employed to set expectations for what that looks like, can we truly discover ourselves as spiritually mature. In the meantime, essays like this (and a practice with the mushrooms) may help along the way.

CHAPTER 21

The Prophetic State and the DMT Effect

The Hebrew Bible as the Source for a Theoneurological Model of Spiritual Experience

by Rick Strassman

At the end of *DMT: The Spirit Molecule* (2001), in which I describe the clinical DMT research that took place at the University of New Mexico in the early 1990s, I was left with several unanswered questions concerning the nature of the DMT world: Where is it? What does it consist of? Why should we interact with it? While grappling with those questions a higher order problem emerged: the need for a better model that could incorporate features of the DMT experience than those I originally brought to bear on my study. My solution to the latter problem, which provides solutions to the former ones, has been to adopt the model of prophetic experience articulated in the Hebrew Bible as a comprehensive and cogent system by which to model the DMT effect. This is the topic of my new book, *DMT and the Soul of Prophecy* (2014).

My definition of 'prophecy' is any spiritual experience described as occurring in a Biblical figure—visions, voices, out of body experiences, extreme emotions, novel insights. This differs from the contemporary popular definition of prophecy as 'predicting.' Foretelling may occur in Biblical prophetic experience, but is not required for the definition. Many prophetic figures never foretold events, those who made predictions in a prophetic state were often wrong, and false prophets may make accurate predictions. In addition, one may predict by other means, such as weather forecasts via deductive reasoning.

Prophecy became associated with foretelling because of how the Greek translation of the Hebrew Bible (the first translation from its original

Hebrew) rendered the Hebrew word for "prophet." The Hebrew word is *navi*, derived from a three letter root which means: to communicate, utter, interpret, act as a spokesman, and similar notions. However, the Greeks placed great emphasis on foretelling in their seeking of spiritual experiences. We see this in their notion of 'divination,' equating communing with the divine and seeing into the future. The Greek translation of *navi* is *prophētes*, meaning one who 'speaks before'; that is, speaks about a thing before it happens. Here we see a powerful example of how 'all translation is interpretation.'

My interest in performing clinical psychedelic drug research grew out of an interest in the biology of spiritual experience. I was an undergraduate when the widespread influx of both Eastern religious meditation practices and psychedelic drugs was fully underway. Both technologies provided reliable access to highly altered states of consciousness. In listening to and reading accounts of the experiences wrought by both, I was struck by phenomenological similarities between the two states. This overlap suggested to me the notion of a similar biological brain state occurring in both sets of experiences. I wondered if a particular area in the brain might be activated by psychedelic drugs and meditation. Once activated, this "spirit gland" would affect the function of other brain sites mediating the perceptual, cognitive, emotional, and other hallmark alterations in consciousness. I learned about the pineal gland and its venerated role in esoteric spiritual 'physiologies.' Diagrams of Kabbalistic *sefirot* and Hindu *chakras* pointed to the area associated with the pineal gland as being activated by, or responsible for, the highest degree of spiritual attainment.

The pineal gland is a third eye in lower vertebrates, complete with a cornea, retina, and lens. It receives light input from the environment and converts it into chemical signals affecting skin color and temperature regulation. The gland migrated inward as vertebrates evolved, and in mammals continues as a light sensor, but only indirectly. Mammalian pineal melatonin regulates seasonal reproduction and other endocrine-related sexual functions. The biological and psychological effects of melatonin in humans were only beginning to be investigated in the mid-1980s at which time I chose to study it as my first research project as an independent investigator. There were some data suggesting highly psychoactive properties of melatonin and I hoped that if it turned out to have psychedelic effects, my search for a 'spirit gland,' and the means by which it exerted those effects, would be over.

It turned out that the psychological effects of melatonin were mild; primarily sedating. While we discovered an important role for melatonin in temperature regulation in humans, I remained focused on the psychedelic questions that had originally motivated the pineal project. By that time I had learned about DMT and turned my attention toward developing a study of this compound in 1988.

After two years of working my way through the US federal bureaucracy that regulates such research, I began my study of DMT. DMT drew my interest because of its endogenous nature—that is, the body makes it, primarily in the lungs. Scientists had determined the presence of DMT in psychedelic plants from Latin America in the late 1940s, but it was not until the mid-1950s that Stephen Szára in Hungary discovered its psychedelic effects in humans. Soon thereafter DMT, 5-MeO-DMT, and bufotenine were found in lower animals. A few years later these findings were extended to human urine and blood samples.

While DMT never attained the popularity of LSD within either the recreational drug use or psychiatric research domains, valuable human studies demonstrated its profoundly psychedelic effects and safety in carefully screened, supervised, and followed-up volunteers. Interestingly, psychiatric research focused on the possible role of DMT in psychosis, rather than more in highly valued altered states of consciousness. Be that as it may, the passage of the Controlled Substances Act in 1970 effectively ended all research with DMT, LSD, and other psychedelics in the U.S. and abroad.

We administered a number of different doses of intravenous DMT to volunteers who were psychiatrically and physically healthy, as well as experienced with psychedelic drugs. Between 1990 and 1995, we administered approximately 400 doses of various strengths of DMT to nearly five dozen volunteers. We generated a tremendous amount of biological data, including cardiovascular, autonomic, and endocrinological.

However, the subjective effects were of most interest to me. We tracked those by careful clinical interviewing as well as paper and pencil test results using a new rating scale—the HRS. Effects began within a couple of heartbeats, peaked at two minutes, and resolved by 30 minutes. Research volunteers described a nearly immediate powerful "rush," a feeling of inner pressure, excitement, anxiety, and acceleration. This climaxed in the dissociation of the mind from the body at the higher doses at which time the awareness of the subject entered into a world of light. The light was preternaturally bright, saturated, and intense. In most cases the kaleidoscopic, buzzing, rapidly morphing geometric patterns coalesced into more recognizable shapes. For more than half of the volunteers these shapes assumed the form of what they described as beings or entities, sentient and powerful interactive presences inhabiting the DMT world.

Early on in the study I encountered a problem intrinsic to the models that I brought to bear on my research. This concerned how I responded to the volunteers' unshakable conviction that what they had just witnessed was as real or more real than everyday reality. The three models were the psychoanalytic, psychopharmacologic, and Zen Buddhist. All three posit the basic unreality of what one apprehends in the DMT state. The psycho-analytic model believes that the visions, voices, and interactions are sym-bolic representations of unconscious psychological conflicts or wishes. The Zen Buddhist model teaches that the visions and voices are psycho-logical detritus being shed by the mind on its way toward the goal of enlightenment—a state without concepts, images, forms, feelings, or any content. The psychopharmacologic model suggests that the brain is gener-ating these experiences in response to the drug. The psychopharmacology approach is nested within that of the reigning paradigm for the scientific investigation of spirituality—*neurotheology*. This model suggests that par-ticular stimuli result in a brain reflex that is later called spiritual, a reflex whose existence serves evolutionarily adaptive functions.

Even unspoken, my assumptions about the 'unreal' nature of what the volunteers were describing could not help but transmit some existential skepticism. However, I was repeatedly told by my subjects that the DMT experience did not feel like a dream or even like any other psychedelic drug effect; volunteers could not accept that the brain simply generated the experience of a level of reality so complex, different, and seemingly real as the DMT world; and much of the content seemed completely unrelated to the psychological concerns of the volunteer. Research participants began being less forthcoming with some of the most interesting aspects of their drug sessions. In response to this I decided to perform a thought experi-ment. I took their reports to be 'true' rather than 'not true.' I could at least temporarily assume the worldview that my research subjects did and we would then be discussing their experiences standing on the same existen-tial platform, as it were. After my study was over I could turn to models that might support such an approach.

I began looking into the notions of dark matter and parallel universes as explanatory models for how the mind-brain complex of the DMT-mod-ified volunteer could be peering into external, objective, freestanding par-allel levels of reality. There is appeal to these theories because they provide a rigorous mechanistic explanation. However, there still remained several issues that a 'scientific' perspective did not address. For example, why was the mind-brain complex configured this way? Why didn't the injection of DMT cause one to grow an extra nose instead of occasioning the impres-sion of being transported to a seemingly alternate level of reality? Another issue absent from discussions of these theories was the nature or value of the information contained in these usually invisible worlds. In other words, what good is obtained from entering into them? In the case of my DMT subjects, the primary realization they returned with was the existence of such realms. However, the information content, and how they would use what they experienced, were less well articulated.

I decided to turn to the other major system of thought that concerns itself with usually invisible worlds—that of religion. In addition to developing methods to attain spiritual experiences and systems to characterize them, religious systems have also labored to extract moral-ethical information/guidelines and theological truths that the solely scientific perspective does not, by definition, address. Buddhism's approach to the reality bases of the DMT world radically differed from the unshakeable conviction of the volunteers, and was for that reason less than ideal. In addition, there was only one "typical" enlightenment-like experience in our dozen volunteers; thus, the DMT state itself wasn't anything like the goal of Buddhist meditation—a unitive-mystical enlightenment state free of a sense of self, absent any content.

Latin American shamanism has become increasingly popular as an explanatory model for the psychedelic drug state, particularly that of DMT as it is the visionary ingredient in ayahuasca. The ethical-moral shortcomings of most Latin American shamans, and the lack of a recognizable Western God in its cosmology and metaphysics (which is also the case with Buddhism) are two major stumbling blocks to widespread acceptance of this model. On the other hand, it does have the advantage of accepting the reality bases of the spiritual worlds and the beings that seem to inhabit it.

A confluence of events led me to return to my Jewish roots and open the Hebrew Bible. One of my motivations was to determine if a cogent spiritual model might exist within this text, revered by half of the world's population. Soon, the notion of a prophetic state of consciousness began to take shape. The more I considered the phenomenon of Biblical prophecy, the more it comported with the reports of my DMT volunteers. The state was highly interactive, full of content, phenomenology, and information. It was experienced as outside of oneself. At the same time, it possessed more of a reality valence than everyday reality—information obtained in that state unquestioningly took precedence in determining how one is to understand reality and interact with it.

As is the case with most secular educated Westerners, I was not especially familiar with the Hebrew Bible (what is commonly referred to as the 'Old' Testament). I was exposed to it as a child but certainly had never turned to it as an adult for either spiritual insights nor as a way to understand the psychedelic drug effect. There are many obstacles to entering into the worldview of the authors of the Hebrew Bible. One of these is intellectual—what exactly is it saying? The meaning of even its opening line presages the challenges we face in comprehending the text: 'In the beginning God created the heavens and the earth'? Who or what is 'God'? 'The beginning' of what? Where did God get the materials with which to "create" the heavens and the earth? What exactly are 'the heavens'?

It was clear that I needed help in reading and grasping the meaning of the text, and subsequently discovered the medieval Jewish philosophers and commentators who lived and wrote between approximately 800-1750 CE. These figures include Maimonides, Abraham ibn Ezra, Nachmanides, Saadiah, and Spinoza. Technically, Spinoza did not live during the medieval period, but his writings represented the end of a particularly medieval way of approaching the Hebrew Bible.

Along with my two Hebrew-English dictionaries, the English translations of these authors' commentaries were indispensable to understand the plain meaning of the Biblical text. However, it was not simply the words that they helped explicate but the actual narratives the words described. In addition, they used common sense and the science of their time to interpret the narratives—what they say about the nature of God, nature, human nature, society, and history.

Another level of resistance to delving into the Hebrew Bible is its use of the word 'God' to represent divinity. In my case, I performed a similar thought experiment to that which allowed me a deeper access to my volunteers' reports of their DMT experiences. I decided to accept the possibility that God existed. That way, I could explore where such a notion might possibly lead. My Buddhist background provided the first toehold upon which I could base my belief in God.

I had always wondered about cause and effect as taught by Buddhism to be eternal and value-free. How could cause and effect be eternal if nothing else was? Impermanence of all phenomena is one of the fundamental tenets taught by the Buddha. In addition, cause and effect did not appear to be value-free. Certain behaviors and thoughts seemed to be encouraged or rewarded whereas others seemed to be discouraged or punished. I wondered about who created and sustains cause-and-effect and who determines the direction that cause and effect takes? Positing the existence, power, will, wisdom, omnipresence, love, and eternality of God solved these problems for me.

One of the most difficult features for readers of the Hebrew Bible to accommodate is its descriptions of God's 'personality' and 'behavior.' There is a term—'anthropomorphism'—that refers to attributing human characteristics to nonhuman forces and processes. If a human did something that hurt us or made us feel special, we would consider her/him as being angry or loving. People are only able to understand terms with which they are familiar and most of us are mostly familiar with how things work at the human level. When the text refers to God 'punishing,' it is an anthropomorphic way of describing a particular case of cause-and-effect. For example, the Hebrew Bible prescribes particular agricultural practices as 'handed down' by God, the abrogation of which results in famine, war, pestilence, and exile. These plagues are the result of cause and effect—over-farming, excessive use of pesticides, greed over boundary lines—that then result in certain consequences. These consequences, if executed by a person, would be seen as punishment.

Prophetic figures in the Hebrew Bible are male and female, handsome and unattractive, young and old, from the ruling class and the common folk—they range throughout the entire gamut of society. The text also describes some exigencies which may make prophecy more likely, such as ecstasy, sensory deprivation, certain locations, and nearness to death. There are no explicit references to the use of exogenous psychoactive agents despite suggestions regarding ergot alkaloids, cannabis, and DMT. The presence of endogenous DMT makes such speculation unnecessary. And while it is true that we do not yet know whether endogenous DMT levels rise in association with non-drug spiritual experiences, this is significantly more likely to be the case than a conclusive determination of the use of exogenous agents in the Hebrew Bible. More to the point, the search for endogenous agents lends itself to the belief that if only we found the plant or substance eliciting prophecy (for the purposes of this discussion), we could also consume it and become prophets.

The Hebrew Bible teaches that prophecy devolves upon someone through the will of God. God decides who will experience prophecy, the content of the prophetic state, the phenomenology the state is transmitting, and the interpretation of the message. God is the source of prophecy and interacting with God or God's intermediaries/angels is the goal of prophecy. Even in the case of spiritual practices, these simply increase one's readiness to receive communication from God rather than bringing prophecy on as such—there is no guarantee.

The majority of my new book compares the phenomenology of the DMT and the prophetic states. In this project, I begin by using the default position of the DMT experience as explicated by the Buddhist psychological categorization of components of mental experience that I used to develop the HRS rating scale. These include physical sensations, cognitive effects on thought processes and content, emotional effects, modifications of will and volition, and perceptual effects. I carefully reviewed the Hebrew Bible for every description of prophetic experience and placed examples of, say, visual effects into the 'perception' category. I did the same for emotional, cognitive, and other variations in consciousness that prophetic figures report. The overlap in phenomenology is striking, especially regarding perceptual effects, visual ones in particular.

In reviewing the phenomenology found in both states, a new category emerged which I called 'relatedness.' This encompasses the nature of the interactions occurring between the experient and the DMT or prophetic world. There may be a healing interaction taking place, arguing and negotiating, and other dynamics that the pre-existing categories did not adequately capture. In comparing descriptions of relatedness between the DMT and prophetic states, I began noticing that the prophetic state appeared significantly richer and more varied than the DMT one. As the imparting of information is the most important role of relatedness, this led me to assess the relationship between the prophetic and DMT messages.

In comparing message content, my default position was reversed. I first developed categories of the prophetic message—such as morality/ethics, information about God, predictions of the future, and reward and punishment. I then reviewed my DMT notes and binned examples of, say, ethical information into the Biblical category so-labeled. Here again, the preponderance of data was contained in the prophetic rather than the DMT state. That is to say, the DMT state appeared aesthetics-rich but information-poor whereas the prophetic state was at least as aesthetically rich but overwhelmingly more information-rich.

The medievalists' metaphysics of how prophecy works takes into account this disparity in information content but with more or less equivalency regarding phenomenology. Their theories hinge on the Aristotelian separation of the mind into rational and imaginative faculties. The imaginative faculty is the area in which corporeal elements of the mind are manifest, including feelings, somatic effects, and perceptions. The rational faculty deals with abstract formless ideas, and because of its incorporeal currency, is believed to be closer to God who is similarly invisible and incorporeal. In the metaphysics of prophecy, it is believed that the influence of God and/or God's intermediaries overflow onto the rational and imaginative faculties. The rational faculty more or less accurately translates the phenomenological contents of the imaginative faculty into ideas and words that can be understood and communicated.

The medievalists discuss the notion of being 'qualified' for prophecy. This means having equally and highly developed rational and imaginative faculties. The state of the imaginative faculty, the more corporeal, is a result of nature and nurture, whereas the rational faculty can be developed to an even higher degree through education. Being qualified is no guarantee, however, of attaining prophecy, but does make it more likely if the situation calls for it.

In this model, one can suggest that DMT is primarily affecting the imaginative faculty but not the rational one. In prophecy, I am proposing that divine overflow may increase the activity of endogenous DMT 'from above.' In the clinical research situation, DMT 'from below' is activating the imaginative faculty. Prophecy thus differs from the DMT state, to the extent that DMT may be involved in imaginative function, with respect to the source of the elevation of DMT and the lack of an effect on the rational faculty by DMT. It is possible that exogenous DMT would increase one's 'qualifications' for prophecy by increasing the activity of the imaginative faculty. However, without a correspondingly well-developed and activated rational faculty—and the decision by God to bestow prophecy—the experience is simply that of a stimulated imagination. This would also be the case if this hypothetical elevation of DMT activity is self-induced through spiritual practices—which is also hypothetical at this point.

These considerations are the bases of the new model I propose for understanding the relationship between the brain-mind complex and the spiritual experience. I have labelled this new model *theoneurology* in order to distinguish it from neurotheology. In the latter model, a biological reflex in the brain generates the impression of communicating with God. In theoneurology, God uses the brain-mind complex as the agent by means of which the communication in reality takes place. These two models are meant to be complementary, rather than antagonistic, as they are approaching the same phenomena occurring in the same mind-brain matrix. One is a bottom-up approach while the other is top-down. One explicates the fine-tuned mechanisms whereas the other offers a more abstract but ethical-moral theocentric model of causality and metaphysics.

The use of psychedelics for spiritual purposes is being investigated in clinical research as well as being practically utilized in the larger community. One consequence of considering the implications of a Hebrew Bible-based theoneurological model in clinical research is to extend the notion of spiritual experience beyond that of the mystical unitive state into the more interactive relational one that occurs in response to DMT and is so well-documented in the Hebrew Bible.

In the non-academic environment, one may consider the Hebrew Bible as a key to understanding and integrating his/her psychedelic drug experiences. It may be that the concepts, images, vocabulary, narratives, and messages of the Hebrew Bible provide a more suitable model for understanding and integrating the contemporary Western psychedelic drug experience than Eastern religious and Latin American shamanic ones. And those who now read and revere the Hebrew Bible may consider the judicious entry into a pharmacologically-induced state of heightened imaginative activity in order to resonate more deeply with the mind out of which the prophetic text emerged.

CHAPTER 22

'It is so Beautiful'

The Role of Psychedelics in Post-Apartheid South Africa

by About Yellow

It's a big fat continent this, bloated like a tic and it ain't my home this burning lump of land but I like it well enough and, damn, sometimes I even love it, this Africa. And it's an interesting place in terms of drugs because this is the cradle of humanity, where we all hark back to. And there are Bushmen and Sangomas, high and wise with the medicines of the land, the Bufane, Malpitta and Khat.

There are cities and towns and a suburbia dull with the monotone of Christianity and daytime TV, and other cities exploding out of their own ribcages with the exuberance of mushrooms and alcohol. And there is also, undeniably, a race division at play and it's that which concerns me here. Why, for example, are psychedelics seen mainly as white culture drugs and what role could they have in breaking down unhealthy dynamics between individuals?

It's hard to talk in general because there are so many perspectives and worlds even within a few miles or apartment strata of each other. So here's a subjective narrative about Ernest, the Malawian bloke, who laboured on a farm where I worked just outside Cape Town. Sometimes we shared a joint together but only when the white Afrikaans family who owned the farm were away. Not that they didn't like weed, far from it, these where full-moon-meditation hippies and smoked with me often. But there's an invisible graphene curtain between owner and labourer, a division that is almost always a white/black division. It is in fact hard to differentiate these two intimate elements of the South African's political and personal landscape.

Class and race are very closely linked and in many examples the dynamic between individuals seems assignable to class inequalities and expectations more than anything else. Often people are cognitively non-racial in their thinking or attitudes but none-the-less play out ingrained behaviour patterns based on the roles of employer and employee, family and maid, farmer and labourer.

It isn't necessarily easy to break down people's fear of over-stepped boundaries. Ernest had, for a short time, insisted on calling me 'madam' for example. We were doing very similar work and being paid roughly the same amount but I was a traveller with my own money and an English middle-class background, education and confidence. We were negotiating a class/cultural difference over and above a racial one. For better or worse, it was also largely me that dictated the terms of that negotiation. I rejected his version of us in favour of my own more comfortable one when I suggested he drop the 'madam' and call me by my name.

Being able to be high together was an important part of that new relationship. The sharing of work or food are two of the things that most successfully bring about co-operation and appreciation, even if that is through nothing more than necessity. But it is through shared emotional experiences (be them spiritual, transcendental or purely recreational) that real understanding and even love can be born.

It should have been a great opportunity to get to know each other better when Ernest found my mushrooms one night and asked if we could take them. But at that point it was a strange formal closeness between us, full of clumsy disregarded etiquettes and language difficulties and he had never heard of any drug beyond the black ash weed you get in the townships.

I tried my best to explain what they were and how they might affect him. I couldn't talk about the Sixties or the Nineties or any of the literature or films. Instead I mimed flying and contoured my face into something like peace and smiled. That's what these mushrooms in this bag make you feel, I was saying. He was confused but up for it. The guy drinks almost to destruction and is up for anything. Young, reckless and pushing at life, I think it's why we were friends, our point of reference in each other. But I said no to taking the mushrooms. Christ, it was late already and we had to be up at 6am for work. I also said no again to taking them at the weekend and the question began to haunt me; was I saying no to taking them with him *at all* and, if so, why?

It feels like the uncomfortable answer might have something to do with my being protective. I don't want to be the women who introduced alcohol to the Native Americans and, hell, Ernest ain't got a background, or friendship group, or cultural experience for something like this. He lives in a tin shanty with a stick under his bed to scare off the prostitutes who come singing at his door like mermaids after dark. Set and setting are not that idyllic at his end of town.

It had been many weeks of inward raging watching Ernest and my host mother on the farm. It'd been 'yes madam, yes madam' all day long for too many days; treated like a kid but acts like one too. That's the bit of this whole race relation thing people forget to mention, that it's a dynamic played out by two people at a time. And it's no good the white Afrikaans lady or the black man alone pushing for change. She has to change her role along with him if that long held comfort blanket of 'madam' is to be dropped. So I hated them both at times. Ernest, bowing himself out of respect with every fawning subjugation. And she, rainbow warrior star child and self-modelled hippie with all the one-love tripped up trappings and concepts, keeping that man a school boy.

But there was I withholding the drugs from him, teacher-like. Sure I was simply performing the role he had helped put me in by asking permission to take them rather than assuming his right. But that ain't really an excuse. So in the end, that was my decision, I gave them to him on my last day at the place. And I gave him my mobile number too and I said 'call me afterwards, I want to know all about it'. It was his responsibility now.

Thirty-six hours after I left the glaring, too bright, Eastern Cape I get a call. It's the middle of the night and I'm in a field. *Darkness*. And it's Ernest talking slow and loud because his English ain't so good on the phone and our signal is weak. 'Hello my love,' he says. 'It is so beautiful.' And that was it. The line broke up and he flew away. But I was no longer 'madam', he had granted me the title of 'love', and I revelled in it.

So what's my point here? Well I guess I'm questioning why a drug that can have such a beautiful effect remains exclusively part of white drug culture, while the crack and the crystal meth and the Mandrax are associated with the black world. It does feel like an easy situation to draw a conspiracy out of. Rumours and evidence abound that the apartheid era government in South Africa introduced Mandrax to the black population of Cape Town, in order to keep them conveniently doped and pliant. Other drugs, of course, are not so desirable to governments.

It was the hippies that led the anti-Vietnam protests and LSD, with its propensity to free the mind of establishment ideas, which was held to have a central part in that. Is it an instinctual fear of the liberated black man that holds white culture back from sharing her drugs? I don't know. What I do know is that class and cultural differences are deeply ingrained into drug culture and the seat of all a psychedelic taker's references are Western, even if the drugs they take are not. And like a work of literature, or a painting, a drug is embedded in the historical and cultural context of its author, reader and user.

So to my mind there is a role for psychedelics in helping to transform South Africa's many cultural landscapes but only in so far as they can help us all individually to break the personal dynamics and roles we all live within, to make us more consciously aware of our performance and how we might reconstruct our relationships with each other. Be that with our parents, our lovers or the colleagues that call us 'madam'.

References

Taboo from the Jungle to the Clinic by Rev. Nemu
1. Frecska, E et al. *Enhancement of Creative Expression and Entopic Phenomena as After-Effects of Repeated Ayahuasca Ceremonies* –, JoPD 44:3 191–199 (Frescka A)
2. Schmid J. T. et al. *Subjective Theories about (Self-)Treatment with Ayahuasca – Anthropology of Consciousness* Vol. 21, Issue 2, pp 188–204, Fall 2010
3. RL Carhart-Harris et al. *Psychiatry's next top model: cause for a re-think on drug models of psychosis and other psychiatric disorders* - J Psychopharmacol September 2013 vol. 27 no. 9 771–778
4. Pratt, L. A. et al. *Antidepressant Use in Persons Aged 12 and Over: United States, 2005–2008* - NCHS Data Brief No. 76, October 2011
5. Pers. Comm. – And I'm not telling you who said it, sorry!
6. Frecska, Ede. *The Risks and Potential Benefits of Ayahuasca Use from a Psychopharmacological Perspective* - in *The Internationalization of Ayahuasca* (Labate & Jungaberle, eds) p. 165
7. Frecska, Ede. *The Risks and Potential Benefits of Ayahuasca Use from a Psychopharmacological Perspective* - in *The Internationalization of Ayahuasca* (Labate & Jungaberle, eds)
8. Callaway, J. C., Grob, C.S. 1998. *Ayahuasca preparations and serotonin reuptake inhibitors: a potential combination for severe adverse interactions.* -. JoPD, 30:367–369.
9. Schmid J. T. et al. *Subjective Theories about (Self-)Treatment with Ayahuasca – Anthropology of Consciousness* Vol. 21, Issue 2, pp 188–204, Fall 2010
10. 10Tupper, K. W. *Entheogenic Healing: The spiritual effects and therapeutic potential of ceremonial ayahausca use* -. in *The healing power of spirituality: How faith helps humans thrive* - J. H. Ellens (ed.), (vol. 3, pp. 269–282) (Westport, CT: 2009).
11. Beyer, S. *On the Origin of Ayahuasca* - http://www.singingtotheplants.com/2012/04/on-origins-of-ayahuasca/
12. *Ibid.*
13. Simson, A. 1886 *Travels in the wilds of Ecuador, and the exploration of the Putamayo River*. London. 178
14. *Ibid.* 181

15. Ethan Watters 2010. *Crazy Like Us: The Globalization of the American Psyche*. New York: 77
16. *Ibid.* 100
17. http://callicott.blogspot.co.uk/2014/04/el-congreso-nierika.html
18. Chalker-Scott, Linda. 2004. *The Myth of Biodynamic Agriculture* -, Ph. D, Extension Horticulturist and Associate professor, Washington State University.
19. *Effects of Full-Moon Definition on Psychiatric Emergency Department Presentations* - Varinder S. et al *ISRN Emergency Medicine* Vol. 2014 (2014), Article ID 398791
20. Kristofic, Jim. 2011. *Navajos Wear Nikes: A Reservation Life.* 146
21. There is a caveat here: I am given bad advice sometimes, during ceremony but not from my sacrament. But by observing conditions, parameters and outcomes over time, one gradually calibrates one's invisible meter to distinguish between different sources offering good and bad advice. In my case, good advice comes gently and unassumingly, usually surprisingly, accompanied by a certain something. Bad advice comes urgently and insistently, but fleetingly. I do not generally receive transmissions involving mathematical manipulations of Chinese divinatory systems.
22. Dickins, Robert. *Psychedelic Press UK.* 2014
23. This raises a traditional taboo, which is an aversion towards sharing ayahuasca visions. Daimistas in Brazil discuss their visions only in exceptional circumstances, and the same has been reported in the indigenous world. Any Western-trained talking therapist collecting accounts should take pains to understand the logic behind this taboo first.
24. Protocol at http://www.maps.org/research/mdma/MP8_amend4_final_7Feb2012web.pdf
25. *Alterations in brain and immune function produced by mindfulness meditation* – Davidson RJ, et al. *Psychosomatic Medicine.* 2003; 65: 564–70
26. *Singing to the Plants: A Guide to Mestizo Shamanism in the Upper Amazon* - Stephan V, Beyer, (New Mexico, 2009) chapter 5.
27. Newton, I. 1687. *Principia mathematica*
28. Narby, J. *Shamans and scientists*: www.deoxy.org.shamansci.htm
29. Callicott, Christina. 2013. *Interspecies communication in the Western Amazon: Music as a form of conversation between plants and people* - *European Journal of Ecopsychology* 4: 32–43
30. Hornborg, Alf. 2001. *Vital Signs: And ecosemiotic perspective on the human ecology of Amazonia* –in *Sign Systems Studies* Vol. 29.1. Tartu. 121
31. Frecska, Ede. *The Risks and Potential Benefits of Ayahuasca Use from a Psychopharmacological Perspective* - in *The Internationalization of Ayahuasca* (Labate & Jungaberle, eds). 151
32. Pregnancy-info.net
33. Bustos, Susana. 2010. *Icaros: Song and Healing in Ayahuasca Ceremonies*: Talk given at MAPS: Psychedelic Science in the 21st Century. https://vimeo.com/15751555

No Imperfection in the Budded Mountain by Andy Roberts

1. The Telegraph. *"Marvellous McGough"*. 14 April, 2013. http://www.telegraph.co.uk/culture/books/3649049/The-marvellous-McGough.html
2. Cunliffe, Dave. 1991. *Blackburn Brainswamp*. Bradford. Redbeck Press. 23
3. Miles, Barry. 2010. *Allen Ginsberg Beat Poet*. London. Virgin Books. 259
4. PlosBlogs. *"The Plot to Turn On the World: The Leary/Ginsberg Acid Conspiracy"*. 14 April 2013: http://blogs.plos.org/neurotribes/2011/04/21/the-plot-to-turn-on-the-world-the-learyginsberg-acid-conspiracy/
5. Sinclair, Iain. 1971. *The Kodak Mantra Diaries*. London. Albion Village Press.
6. Maschler, Tom. 2005. *Publisher*. London. Picador. 280
7. Ibid.
8. Sinclair, Iain. 2006. *The Kodak Mantra Diaries*. Coventry. Beat Scene. 87 (re-print of 1971 edition with Postscript by Sinclair.)
9. Maschler, Tom. 2005. *Publisher*. London. Picador. 281
10. Ginsberg, Allen. 1968. *Wales Visitation*. London. Cape Goliard.
11. Maschler, Tom. 2005. *Publisher*. London. Picador. 281
12. Sinclair, Iain. 2006. *The Kodak Mantra Diaries*. Coventry. Beat Scene. 56 (re-print of 1971 edition with Postscript by Sinclair.)
13. Ginsberg, Allen. 1994. *Holy Soul Jelly Roll* (booklet to accompany CD box set). Rhino Word Beat R271693). 21
14. Ibid.
15. Sinclair, Iain. 2002. *Landor's Tower*. London. Granta. 87
16. Portuges, Paul Cornel. 1981. *The Visionary Poetics of Allen Ginsberg*. San Diego: Blue Pacific Books. 122
17. Sinclair, Iain. 2006. *The Kodak Mantra Diaries*. Coventry. Beat Scene. 70 (re-print of 1971 edition with Postscript by Sinclair.)
18. Firing Line. WOR-TV, 3 September 1968. http://www.youtube.com/watch?v=eKBAJYceQ54
19. Ginsberg, Allen. 1994. *Holy Soul Jelly Roll*. Rhino Word Beat R271693
20. Wales OnLine. 14 April, 2003. *'For sale: Allen Ginsberg poem written while on drugs in Wales'*: http://www.walesonline.co.uk/news/wales-news/sale-allen-ginsberg-poem-written-2494407

Psychedelic Trickster by David Luke

1. Adler, G. 1976. *C.G. Jung letters: Volume 2, 1951–1961*. London. Routledge & Kegan Paul.
2. Luke, D. 2011. Experiential reclamation and first person parapsychology. *Journal of Parapsychology*. 75. 185–199
3. Lee, M. A., & Shlain, B. 1985. *Acid dreams: The complete social history of LSD: The CIA, the sixties, and beyond*. New York. Grove Press.
4. Stevens, J. 1988. *Storming Heaven: LSD and the American dream*. London. William Heinemann. 198
5. Black, D. 2001. *Acid: A new secret history of LSD*. London. Vision Paperbacks. 51
6. Krippner, S. 2006. Personal communication, January 19.

7. Horn, S. 2009. *Unbelievable: Investigations into ghosts, poltergeists, telepathy, and other unseen phenomena, from the Duke parapsychology laboratory.* New York. Ecco Press.
8. Black, D. 2001. *Acid:A new secret history of LSD.* London. Vision Paperbacks. 53
9. *Ibid.*
10. Black, D. Acid. 2001. A new secret history of LSD. London. Vision Paperbacks. 73
11. Black, D. Acid. 2001. A new secret history of LSD. London. Vision Paperbacks.

Watts Ego by Robert Dickins

1. Evans-Wentz, WY. 2011. *The Fairy Faith in Celtic Countries.* Glastonbury. Lost Library. 468–469
2. Leary et al. 2008. *The Psychedelic Experience.* London. Penguin Classics. 72
3. Huxley, Aldous. 1994. *The Doors of Perception and Heaven and Hell.* Flamingo. 32
4. *Ibid.*
5. Huxley, Aldous. 1994. *The Doors of Perception and Heaven and Hell.* Flamingo. 6
6. Huxley, Aldous. 1999. *Moksha.* Rochester. Park Street Press. 256
7. Huxley, Aldous. 1962. *Island.* London. Chatto & Windus. 137
8. Watts, Alan. 1962 (2013). *The Joyous Cosmology.* Novato. New World Library. 81
9. Watts, Alan. 1962 (2013). *The Joyous Cosmology.* Novato. New World Library. 42
10. Watts, Alan. 1962 (2013). *The Joyous Cosmology.* Novato. New World Library. 76
11. Watts, Alan. 1962 (2013). *The Joyous Cosmology.* Novato. New World Library. 72
12. Watts, Alan. 1962 (2013). *The Joyous Cosmology.* Novato. New World Library. 84
13. Watts, Alan. 1962 (2013). *The Joyous Cosmology.* Novato. New World Library. 88
14. Watts, Alan. 1962 (2013). *The Joyous Cosmology.* Novato. New World Library. 86

Psychedelic Research by Stanislav Grof

1. Vondráček, V. *Farmakologie duše* (Pharmacology of the Soul). Prague: Lékařské knihkupectví a nakladatelství. 1935
2. Nevole, S. *O čtyřrozměrném viděni: Studie z fysiopathologie smyslu prostorového, se zvláštním zřetelem k experimentálníotravě mezkalinem* (Apropos of Four-Dimesional Vision:Study of Physiopathology of the Spatial Sense with Special Regard to Experimental Intoxication with Mescaline. Prague: Lékařské knihkupectví a nakladatelství. 1947

3. Beringer, K. *Der Meskalinrausch* (Mescaline Intoxication). Berlin. Springer. 1927
4. Stoll, W. A. *LSD, ein Phantastikum aus der Mutterkorngruppe.* Schweiz.Arch. Neurol. Psychiat. 60:279. 1947
5. Jung, C. G. *The Archetypes and the Collective Unconscious.* Collected Works, vol. 9,1. Bollingen Series XX, Princeton, N.J.: Princeton University Press. 1959
6. Grof, S. *Psychology of the Future: Lessons from Modern Consciousness Research.* Albany, NY: State University of New York (SUNY) Press. 2000
7. Grof, S. *LSD Psychotherapy.* Sarasota, FL: MAPS Publications. 2001
8. Cohen, S. *LSD and the Anguish of Dying.* Harper's Magazine 231:69,77. 1965
9. Kast, E. C. and Collins, V. J. *LSD and the Dying Patient.* Chicago Med. School Quarterly 26:80. 1966
10. Grof, S. *The Ultimate Journey: Consciousness and the Mystery of Death.* Sarasota, FL.: MAPS Publications. 2006
11. Roubíček, J. *Experimentální psychózy* (Experimental Psychoses). Prague: Statní zdravotnické nakladatelství. 1961
12. Forte, R (ed). *Entheogens and the Future of Religion.* San Francisco: Council on Spiritual Practices. 1997
13. Roberts, T. B. (ed.) *Psychoactive Sacramentals: Essays on Entheogens and Religion.* San Francisco: Council on Spiritual Practices. 2001
14. Grof, S. *The Cosmic Game: Explorations of the Frontiers of Human Consciousness.* Albany, N.Y.: State University New York Press. 1998
15. Pahnke W. *Drugs and mysticism: An analysis of the relationship between psychedelic drugs and themystical consciousness.*Thesis presented to the President and Fellows of Harvard University for the Ph.D. in Religion and Society. 1963
16. Griffiths, R.R., Richards, W. A., McCann, U., and Jesse, R. *Psilocybin can Occasion Mystical Experiences Having Substantial and Sustained Personal Meaning and Spiritual Significance.* Psychopharmacology 187:3, pp. 268–283. 2006
17. Cohen, S. *Lysergic Acid Diethylamide: Side Effects and Complications.* Journal of Nervous and Mental Diseases 130:30. 1960
18. Capra, F. *The Tao of Physics.* Berkeley: Shambhala Publications. 1975
19. Goswami, A. *The Self-Aware Universe.* Los Angeles: J. P. Tarcher. 1995
20. Bohm, D. *Wholeness and the Implicate Order.* London: Routledge & Kegan Paul. 1980
21. Pribram, K. *Languages of the Brain.* Englewood Cliffs, N.J.: Prentice Hall. 1971
22. Prigogine, I. *From Being to Becoming: Time and Complexity in the Physical Sciences.* San Francisco, CA: W.H. Freeman. 1980
23. Sheldrake, R. *A New Science of Life.* Los Angeles: J. P. Tarcher. 1981
24. Wilber, K. *A Theory of Everything: An Integral Vision for Business, Politics, Science and Spirituality.* Berkeley: Shambhala Publications. 2000

The LSD Trial by Toby Slater

1. Blake, W. 2012. 'London' from *The Poetry of William Blake*.
2. Blake, W. 2012. 'The Marriage of Heaven and Hell' from *The Poetry of William Blake*.
3. Shulgin, A. 1995. *PIHKAL: A Chemical Love Story*.
4. Carhart-Harris, R; Leech, R; Hellyer, P.J; Shanahan, M; Feilding, A; Tagliazucchi, E; Chialvo, D.R; Nutt, D: 'The Entropic Brain: A Theory of Conscious States Informed by Neuro-imaging Research with Psychedelic Drugs'.
5. Huxley, A. 1954. *The Doors of Perception*.
6. Hofmann, A. 2008.*Hofmann's Elixir: LSD and the New Eleusis*.
7. Carhart-Harris, R; Leech, R; Hellyer, P.J; Shanahan, M; Feilding, A; Tagliazucchi, E; Chialvo, D.R; Nutt, D: 'The Entropic Brain: A Theory of Conscious States Informed by Neuro-imaging Research with Psychedelic Drugs'.
8. Grof, S. 1992. *The Holotropic Mind*.
9. Campbell, J. 1947. *The Hero With a Thousand Faces*.
10. Campbell, J. 2007. *Practical Campbell: Mysteries Sacred and Profane.*

Archaidelics by Tim Read

1. 1 Jung, Carl. *Collected Works Volume 8*. Routledge and Kegan, Paul. 1969. 414
2. Dass, Ram. *The Only Dance There Is*. Anchor Books. New York 1974. 15
3. Fadiman, Jim. *The Psychedelic Explorer's Guide*. Park Street Press 2011. 198
4. Jeans, James. *The Mysterious Universe*. Cambridge 1930. 134
5. Bohm, David. *Wholeness and the Implicate Order*. Ark. 1980
6. Huxley, Aldous. *The Doors of Perception*. Flamingo 1954. 12–13
7. Campbell, Joseph. *The Hero with a Thousand Faces*. New World Library. 2008.
8. Tarnas, Rick. *Cosmos and Psyche*. Viking 2006. 81
9. Read, Tim. *Walking Shadows*. Muswell Hill Press. 2014
10. Easwaran, Ecknath. *The Bhagavad Gita*. Nilgiri 1985. 2
11. Grof, Stanislav. *The Psychology of the Future*. SUNY press. 2000
12. Waterfield, Robin. *Plato: The Republic*. Oxford University Press. 1993

The Epilogenic Model by Dave King

1. Buschman, T. J., & Miller, E. K. 2007. Top-Down Versus Bottom-Up Control of Attention in the Prefrontal and Posterior Parietal Cortices. *Science, 315* (5820), 1860–1862.
2. Goldstein, D.S, Ross, R.S., & Brady, J.V. 1977. Biofeedback heart rate training during exercise. *Biofeedback and Self-Regulation*, 2, 107–125.
3. Nakao M, Yano E, Nomura S, Kuboki T. 2003 Blood pressure-lowering effects of biofeedback treatment in hypertension: a meta-analysis of randomized controlled trials. *Hypertens Res*. 2003;26:37–46.
4. Peniston EG, Kulkosky PJ. 1989 'Alpha-theta brainwave training and beta-endorphin levels in alcoholics.'. *Alcoholism: Clinical and Experimental Research* 13 (2): 271–279.

5. Linden DE, Habes I, Johnston SJ, Linden S, Tatineni R, Subramanian L, Sorger B, Healy D, Goebel R. 2012 'Real-time self-regulation of emotion networks in patients with depression.'. *PLoS ONE* 7 (6).

6. Tan G, Thornby J, Hammond DC, Strehl U, Canady B, Arnemann K, Kaiser DA. 2009 'Meta-analysis ofEEG biofeedback in treating epilepsy.'. *Journal of Clinical EEG & Neuroscience* 40 (3): 173–179.

7. Kox, M., Stoffels M., Smeekens S.P., van Alfen N., Gomes M., Eijsvogels T.M., Hopman M.T., vander Hoeven J.G., Netea M.G., Pickkers P. 2012. The influence of concentration/meditation on autonomic nervous system activity and the innate immune response: a case study. *Psychosom Med.* 2012 Jun;74(5):489–94.

8. Kox, M., van Eijk, L.T., Zwaag, J., van den Wildenberg, J., Sweep, F., van der Hoeven, J.G.,Pickkers, P. 2014. Voluntary activation of the sympathetic nervous system and attenuation of the innate immune response in humans. PNAS. May 20, 2014 vol. 111 no. 20 7379–7384.

9. Weiss, B. 2004. *Messages from the Masters* (4 ed.). London: Piatkus Books.

10. Grof, S. 2008. *LSD Psychotherapy* (4th ed.). Ben Lomond: MAPS.

11. Metzner, R. 2009. *MindSpace and TimeStream.* Berkeley: Regent Press.

12. Grof, S. 2008. *LSD Psychotherapy* (4th ed.). Ben Lomond: MAPS.

13. Grof, S. 2008. *LSD Psychotherapy* (4th ed.). Ben Lomond: MAPS. 208

14. McElroy, S. L., & Keck, P. E. 1995. Recovered memory therapy: False memory syndrome and other complications. *Psychiatric Annals , 25* (12), 731–735.

15. Leary, T. M., Metzner, R. 1992. *The Psychedelic Experience: A Manual based on the Tibetan Book of the Dead* (2nd ed.). New York: Citadel.

16. Grof, S. 2008. *LSD Psychotherapy* (4th ed.). Ben Lomond: MAPS. 11

17. Grof, S. 2008. *LSD Psychotherapy* (4th ed.). Ben Lomond: MAPS. 281

18. Leary, T. M., Metzner, R. 1992. *The Psychedelic Experience: A Manual based on the Tibetan Book of the Dead* (2nd ed.). New York: Citadel.

19. Krupitsky EM, Burakov AM, Dunaevsky IV, Romanova TN, Slavina TY, Grinenko AY. 2007. Single versus repeated sessions of ketamine-assisted psychotherapy for people with heroin dependence. J Psychoactive Drugs 39: 13–9.

20. Thomas, G., Lucas, P., Capler, N.R., Tupper, K.W. & Martin, G. 2013. Ayahuasca-assisted therapy foraddiction: Results from a preliminary observational study in Canada. Current Drug Abuse Reviews, 6(1), 30–42.

21. Johnson, M.W., Garcia-Romeu, A., Cosimano, M.P., Griffiths, R.R. 2014. Pilot study of the 5-HT2AR agonist psilocybin in the treatment of tobacco addiction. J Psychopharmacol November2014 vol. 28 no. 11 983–992.

22. Moreno FA, Wiegand CB, Taitano EK, Delgado PL. 2006. Safety, tolerability, and efficacy of psilocybin in 9 patients with obsessive-compulsive disorder. *J Clin Psychiatry*;67:1735–1740.

23. Roberts, T.B. 1999. Do entheogen-induced mystical experiences boost the immune system? Psychedelics, peak experiences, and wellness. Adv Mind Body Med. 1999 Spring; 15(2):139–47.

24. Weil, A. 2010. *The Future of Psychedelic & Medical Marijuana Research.* From http://www.maps.org/videos/source/video6.html

Femtheogens by Maria Paraspyrou

1. I Gareth S. Hill. 1992. *Masculine and Feminine: The Natural Flow of Opposites in the Psyche.* Shambhala Publications, Inc.
2. *Ibid.*
3. Llewellyn Vaughan-Lee. 2009. *Return of the Feminine and the World Soul.* Golden Sufi Center.
4. Joseph Campbell. 1988. *The Power of Myth.* Bantam Doubleday Dell Publishing Group; Reissue edition (20 Sep 1989)
5. Gareth S. Hill. 1992. *Masculine and Feminine: The Natural Flow of Opposites in the Psyche.* Shambhala Publications, Inc.
6. *Ibid.* 17
7. Marion Woodman and Elinor Dickson. 1996. *Dancing in the Flames: The Dark Goddess in the Transformation of Consciousness.* Shambhala Publications; Reprint edition (5 Nov 1997)
8. Anne Baring. 2013. *The Dream of the Cosmos: a Quest for the Soul.* Archive Publishing.
9. Marion Woodman and Elinor Dickson. 1996. *Dancing in the Flames: The Dark Goddess in the Transformation of Consciousness.* Shambhala Publications; Reprint edition (5 Nov 1997)
10. Llewellyn Vaughan-Lee. 2009. *Return of the Feminine and the World Soul.* Golden Sufi Center.
11. Terence McKenna. 2007. *The Importance of Psychedelics.* [Podcast] Psychedelic Salon by Lawrence "Lorenzo" Hagerty. Number 117. Available from: http://podbay.fm/show/75943437/e/1196309252?autostart=1. [Accessed 06.11.2014]
12. Marion Woodman and Elinor Dickson. 1996. *Dancing in the Flames: The Dark Goddess in the Transformation of Consciousness.* Shambhala Publications; Reprint edition (5 Nov 1997)
13. *Ibid.*
14. C. G. Jung. 1968. 'Archetypes of the Collective Unconscious'. In The Collected Works of C. G. Jung: Vol. 9 Part 1. Second Edition. Routledge: London (p. 19)
15. Marion Woodman and Elinor Dickson. 1996. *Dancing in the Flames: The Dark Goddess in the Transformation of Consciousness.* Shambhala Publications; Reprint edition (5 Nov 1997)
16. *Ibid.*
17. Terence McKenna. 2007. *The Importance of Psychedelics.* [Podcast] Psychedelic Salon by Lawrence "Lorenzo" Hagerty. Number 117. Available from: http://podbay.fm/show/75943437/e/1196309252?autostart=1. [Accessed 06.11.2014]
18. Terence McKenna. 1992. *Food of the Gods: The Search for the Original Tree of Knowledge.* Rider Books.
19. *Ibid.*
20. Terence McKenna. 2007. *The Importance of Psychedelics.* [Podcast] Psychedelic Salon by Lawrence "Lorenzo" Hagerty. Number 117. Available from: http://podbay.fm/show/75943437/e/1196309252?autostart=1. [Accessed 06.11.2014]

21. Ed Vulliamy. 2011. *Ciudad Juarez is all our futures. This is the inevitable war of capitalism gone mad.* The Guardian [Online] 20th of June. Available from: http://www.theguardian.com/commentisfree/2011/jun/20/war-capitalism-mexico-drug-cartels [Accessed: 6th November 2014]

22. Ed Vulliamy. 2011. *Ciudad Juarez is all our futures. This is the inevitable war of capitalism gone mad.* The Guardian [Online] 20th of June. Available from: http://www.theguardian.com/commentisfree/2011/jun/20/war-capitalism-mexico-drug-cartels [Accessed: 6th November 2014]

23. Anne Baring. 2013. *The Dream of the Cosmos: a Quest for the Soul.* Archive Publishing.

24. Marion Woodman and Elinor Dickson. 1996. *Dancing in the Flames: The Dark Goddess in the Transformation of Consciousness.* Shambhala Publications; Reprint edition (5 Nov 1997). (p. 36)

25. Anne Baring. 2013. *The Dream of the Cosmos: a Quest for the Soul.* Archive Publishing.

26. *Ibid.*

27. Llewellyn Vaughan-Lee. 2009. *Return of the Feminine and the World Soul.* Golden Sufi Center.

28. Llewellyn Vaughan-Lee. 2009. *Return of the Feminine and the World Soul.* Golden Sufi Center.

29. Anne Baring. 2013 *The Dream of the Cosmos: a Quest for the Soul.* Archive Publishing.

30. Marion Woodman and Elinor Dickson. 1996 *Dancing in the Flames: The Dark Goddess in the Transformation of Consciousness.* Shambhala Publications; Reprint edition (5 Nov 1997)

31. Llewellyn Vaughan-Lee. 2009. *Return of the Feminine and the World Soul.* Golden Sufi Center.

32. *Ibid.*

Re-habituating Cognition: Interview with Casey Hardison

1. https://www.gov.uk/government/uploads/system/uploads/attachment_data/file/272360/6941.pdf

On the Nature of Psilocybe Folk by Jack Hunter

1. McKenna, T. & McKenna, D. 1975 [1994]. *The Invisible Landscape: Mind, Hallucinogens, and the I Ching.* New York: HarperCollins.

2. Strassman, R. 2001. *DMT: The Spirit Molecule: A Doctor's Revolutionary Research Into the Biology of Near-Death and Mystical Experiences.* Rochester: Park Street Press.

3. Wilson, R.A. 1977 [2000]. *Cosmic Trigger: Final Secret of the Illuminati.* Tempe: New Falcon Publications.

4. Castaneda, C. 1968 [1976]. *The Teachings of Don Juan: A Yaqui Way of Knowledge.* Harmondsworth: Penguin Books Ltd.

5. Luke, D. 2008. 'Disembodied Eyes Revisited: An Investigation into the Ontology of Entheogenic Entity Encounters.' *The Entheogen Review*, Vol. 7, No. 1, pp. 1–9.
6. Jung, C.G. 2007. Psychology and the Occult. London: Routledge.
7. Myers, F.W.H. 1903 [1992]. *Human Personality and its Survival of Bodily Death*. Norwich: Pelegrin Trust.
8. http://www.beckleyfoundation.org/2010/09/14/effects-of-psilocybin-on-cerebral-blood-flow/

Myco-Metaphysics by Peter Sjöstedt-H

1. Ayer on Logical Positivism, *Men of Ideas*, Bryan Magee. BBC. 1978. Available at http://youtu.be/4cnRJGs08hE?t=7m.
2. Ayer, Alfred Jules. What I saw when I was dead. Sunday Telegraph, 28 August 1988. http://philosopher.eu/others-writings/a-j-ayer-what-i-saw-when-i-was-dead/
3. Osorio D, Zylinski S. Cuttlefish vision in camouflage. *Journal of Experimental Marine Biology and Ecology* 2013;447:
4. Healy K, McNally L Ruxtond GD, Cooper N, Jackson AL. Metabolic rate and body size are linked with perception of temporal information. *Animal Behaviour* 2013;86(4). Available at http://www.sciencedirect.com/science/article/pii/S0003347213003060.
5. Nietzsche F. *The Pre-Platonic Philosophers* (Chicago, IL, 2006), pp. 61–2.
6. Encapsulated best in his magnum opus, *Matter and Memory*.

Seismographic Art by Henrik Dahl

1. Johnson, Ken. 2011. *Are You Experienced: How Psychedelic Consciousness Transformed Modern Art*. Munich: Prestel. 8
2. *Ibid.*
3. Masters, Robert E.L. & Houston, Jean (Eds.). 1968. *Psychedelic Art*. New York: Grove Press. 118
4. Larsen, Lars Bang. 2011. *A History of Irritated Material: Psychedelic Concepts in Neo-Avant-Garde Art* (PhD dissertation). Copenhagen: University of Copenhagen. 115
5. Larsen, Lars Bang. 2011. *A History of Irritated Material: Psychedelic Concepts in Neo-Avant-Garde Art* (PhD dissertation). Copenhagen: University of Copenhagen. 33
6. Larsen, Lars Bang. 2002. *Sture Johannesson*. New York: Lukas & Sternberg. 8
7. Caruana, Laurence. 2001. *First Draft of Manifesto of Visionary Art* (retrieved from http://visionaryrevue.com/webtext/manifesto.contents.html)
8. Caruana, Laurence. 2001. *First Draft of Manifesto of Visionary Art* (retrieved from http://visionaryrevue.com/webtext/manifesto.contents.html).

Cultivating the Teacher by James W. Jesso

1. Helminski, Kabir. 2000. *The Knowing Heart*. Shambhala Publications.
2. Helminski, Kabir. 2000. *The Knowing Heart*. Shambhala Publications. 4

3. Jesso, James. 2013. *Decomposing The Shadow.* SoulsLantern Publishing. 51

4. Psychospiritual maturation is the developmental process of learning one's unwounded self and naturally embodying and expressing that unhindered self within one's personality. I use it interchangeably here with 'spiritual maturity'.

5. Helminski, Kabir. 2000. *The Knowing Heart.* Shambhala Publications. 135

6. Helminski, Kabir. 2000. *The Knowing Heart.* Shambhala Publications. 120

7. *Ibid.*

8. For a more in depth look at the energetic dynamics behind the capacity to increase general perception (consciousness expansion), through community experiences, check out my published book *Soundscapes & Psychedelics.* Available at www.soundscapesbook.com

9. Helminski, Kabir. 2000. *The Knowing Heart.* Shambhala Publications. 120

10. Barks, Coleman. 2004 *The Essential Rumi.* HarperOne.

11. *Decomposing The Shadow* discusses the type of experience that can offer the development of spiritual maturity, the experiential characterizes of those types of experiences, as well as perspective and suggestion of how to cultivate these experiences in much more depth.

12. Helminski, Kabir. 2000. *The Knowing Heart.* Shambhala Publications. 120

13. Carhart-Harris, Robin L., *et al.* 'Neural correlates of the psychedelic state as determined by fMRI studies with psilocybin.' *Proceedings of the National Academy of Sciences* 109.6 (2012): 2138–2143.

14. Jesso, James. 2013. *Decomposing The Shadow.* SoulsLantern Publishing. 83

15. This is a potentially dangerous place to be as its lack of normal life applicability can become a self-perpetuating cycle of confusion.

16. Though, a word of warning: if the community one shares their story with is not practicing a life towards spiritual maturity, and those people become the influence for how one integrate their experience, this very same premise of 'spiritual community' may only lead one deeper and deeper into egoic self-delusions of maturity.

Contributors

Dahl, Henrik: Henrik Dahl is a journalist and critic specializing in psychedelic culture. He is the editor of The Oak Tree Review, a webpage featuring interviews and essays on psychedelia and the sixties counterculture. Dahl has also been a guest editor for Swedish literature and art magazine Papi, editing an issue on intoxication. Before becoming a journalist he studied social anthropology and art history at Lund University. Dahl lives in Malmö, Sweden.

Dickins, Robert: Robert is a writer, author and the Editor of the Psychedelic Press. He specializes in cultural history, poetry, and textual explorations of the psychedelic experience. And as well as having a BA Hons in Journalism, Robert also obtained a Masters of Philosophy in English from the University of Exeter. As well as attempting to set-up the UK's premier psychedelic publisher, he is currently working on a new novel, and is about to undertake a PhD.

Gandy, Sam: Sam has a lifelong interest in nature and wildlife, and in more recent years this fascination has extended to mind, consciousness and altered states. He has an academic background in physical geography, ecology and postgraduate entomology. He has been based for a year at the Department of Biology of the University of Leicester in the UK working on ecological river restoration. In 2014 he started a PhD at the University of Aberdeen and James Hutton Institute working on termites and soils in Ethiopia as part of the alter project that is seeking to alleviate rural poverty in parts of Africa, via improving and protecting ecosystem services.

Grof, Stanislav: Stanislav Grof's professional career has covered a period of over 50 years in which his primary interest has been research of the heuristic and therapeutic potential of non-ordinary states of consciousness. This included initially four years of laboratory research of psychedelics - LSD, psilocybin, mescaline, and tryptamine derivatives - (1956-1960) and fourteen years of research of psychedelic psychotherapy. He spent seven of these years (1960-1967) as Principal Investigator of the psychedelic research program at the Psychiatric Research Institute in Prague,

Czechoslovakia. This was followed by seven years of research of psychedelic psychotherapy in the United States. He is also the co-founder of Transpersonal Psychology.

Hardison, Casey: Casey Hardison is an entheogenic activist, unauthorized researcher and psychedelic chemist who is best known for his indefatigable good mood and enormous energy. Casey attended entheogen-related conferences, wrote articles for the *MAPS Bulletin*, *The Entheogen Review*, and contributed to Erowid. After moving to Britain in 2002, Casey chose to fulfill a ten-year spiritual journey to make LSD, in part to make up for the drought caused by a major LSD bust in the United States. He was arrested and convicted of LSD, DMT, and 2C-B manufacture in Britain.

Hunter, Jack: Jack Hunter is a doctoral candidate in the Department of Archaeology and Anthropology at the University of Bristol. His research takes the form of an ethnographic study of contemporary trance and physical mediumship in Bristol, focusing on themes of personhood, performance, altered states of consciousness and anomalous experience. In 2010 he established *Paranthropology: Journal of Anthropological Approaches to the Paranormal*, as a means to promote an interdisciplinary dialogue on issues relating to paranormal beliefs, experiences and phenomena. He is the editor of *Paranthropology: Anthropological Approaches to the Paranormal* (2012) and *Strange Dimensions: A Paranthropology Anthology* (2015, forthcoming), both of which gather some of the best articles from the first four years of the journal. He is the author of *Why People Believe in Spirits, Gods and Magic* (2012), a beginner's introduction to the anthropology of the supernatural, and co-editor with Dr. David Luke of Talking With the Spirits: Ethnographies from Between the Worlds (2014).

Jay, Mike: Mike Jay is an author, historian and curator who has written widely on drugs and their cultures. His books on the subject include *Emperors of Dreams: drugs in the ninenteeth century* and *High Society: mind-altering drugs in history and culture*, which accompanied the exhibition he curated at the Wellcome Collection, London. He has recently worked with Kew Gardens on their *Intoxication Season* (Sept/Oct 2014).

Jesso, James W: James is a Calgary, Alberta-based author, conference speaker, workshop leader, and event coordinator who used psilocybin mushrooms to heal himself from mental illness resulting from substance abuse. His insightful and engaging book *Decomposing the Shadow: Lessons from the Psilocybin Mushrooms* presents a complete conceptual and cognitive model for the psilocybin mushroom experience as it pertains to psychospiritual maturation and the healing of mental emotional wounds.

For more information on James and his work, check out his website: jameswjesso.com

Johnson, Cody: Cody is an intrepid psychonaut and humanist who blogs about consciousness at psychedelicfrontier.com. He loves discovery, despises dogma, and looks forward to the day when all minds are free to explore the frontier within.

Keen, Roger: Roger Keen is a writer, filmmaker and film critic with a special interest in surrealism, counterculture and psychedelia. He has contributed to many award-winning programmes for the BBC, ITV and Channel 4, and his articles, reviews and short stories have appeared in numerous magazines and webzines, including Threads, Critical Wave, Writer's Monthly, The Third Alternative and The Digital Fix. His memoir *The Mad Artist: Psychonautic Adventures in the 1970s* was published in 2010 and other narrative works are in progress.

King, Dave: Dave is the co-founder of Breaking Convention and the UKC Psychedelics Society. He represented the Beckley Foundation at a House of Lords seminar in 2011, and directed the 2012 Shulgin Blotter Art Fundraiser, which generated $21,000 for Sasha Shulgin's medical care. He is the lead editor of the upcoming book *Neurotransmissions: Essays on Psychedelics*, and was a co-editor of *Breaking Convention: Essays on Psychedelics*. He self-published *A Short Introduction to Psychedelics* in 2008, which is currently undergoing editorial revision prior to print with Scriptor Press. He worked at the National University of Singapore Medical School for two years, conducting translational human immunology research on CMV and T-cell senescence.

Luke, David: David Luke is the Senior Lecturer in Psychology at the University of Greenwich where he teaches an undergraduate course on the Psychology of Exceptional Human Experience. His research focuses on transpersonal experiences, anomalous phenomena, and altered states of consciousness, especially via psychedelics. He has published more than 100 academic papers in this area, including three books, most recently *Talking With Spirits: Ethnographies between the Worlds*, with Jack Hunter.

Nemu, Reverend: Danny's academic background is in the History and Philosophy of Medicine. He spent three years living in Brazil learning about the roots of Daime, and is particularly interested in the transpersonal and the spooky side of ayahuasca. He's also an anarchist, an activist, and an optimist. His book *Science Revealed*, Part 1 of the Nemu's End trilogy, examines the limits of rationalism in science, and will shortly be followed by Part 2 *Neuro-Apocalypse*. Despite being ordained over the internet for $30 in order to perform wedding ceremonies for gullible pagans in Japan, he still knows more about scripture than your average priest: nemusend. co.uk

O'Reilly, Louise: Louise is an artist and illustrator working in a wide range of natural history subjects. She teaches Botanical Illustration at Capel Manor College and Forty Hall and is a painting member of the Chelsea Physic Garden Florilegium Society. Recent commissions include an artists's book about the 17th century gardens at Ham House and Fountain's Florilegia, a large-scale architectural glass commission for a new primary health care building in Chester. In 2013 she was the first artist in residence at Borde Hill Garden in West Sussex and in 2014 she was artist in residence at Mottisfont House and Garden in Hampshire. www.lorva.co.uk

Papaspyrou, Maria: Maria, MSc, is a BACP accredited counsellor and psychotherapist. She has worked as a therapist for 13 years, in the fields of mental health and education, alongside her private practice. She has also been contributing to forums like Breaking Convention, Burning Man, and Boom Festival, supporting the re-introduction of psychedelic agents in psychotherapy. Entheogens and Healing have been major reference points of interest for many years. In Psychedelic Science the two are able to join and she explores the sacramental and healing properties of entheogens, and how these can foster development and the growth of human and societal tacit potential.

Read, Tim: Tim is a medical doctor, psychiatrist and psychotherapist based in London. He was Consultant Psychiatrist at the Royal London Hospital for 20 years leading the Crisis Intervention Service and the Emergency Liaison Service. He has trained in psychoanalytic therapy (IGA) and in transpersonal therapy with Stanislav Grof. He is a certified facilitator of Holotropic Breathwork. Tim is co-founder and commissioning editor for Muswell Hill Press and his book *Walking Shadows: Archetype and Psyche in Crisis and Growth* was published in 2014. walkingshadows.tr@gmail. com

Roberts, Andy: Andy Roberts is an historian of Britain's LSD psychedelic culture and author of *Albion Dreaming: A Social History of LSD in Britain*. His other research interests include, listening to music, hill walking, beach combing, reading, landscapes and their mysteries, natural history and paranormal phenomena. Musically, he has been severely influenced and affected by the Grateful Dead and the Incredible String Band among a host of others. He first fell down the rabbit hole in 1972 and has been exploring the labyrinth of passages ever since. His views on the psyche-delic experience are (basically) – You take a psychedelic and you get high. What happens after that is largely the result of set, setting, and dosage.

Salway, Chris: Chris is a consultant psychiatrist living and working in Somerset. His current role is as the community consultant for Mine-head and West Somerset. He also works one afternoon per week at Broadway Addiction Centre, a drug and alcohol rehabilitation unit in Weston-Super-Mare.

Sessa, Ben: Ben is one of the five co-founders of Breaking Convention, the UK's only psychedelic conference, and the author of several novels and non-fiction books, including *The Psychedelic Renaissance*. He is a pediat-ric psychiatrist and is coordinating Britain's first MDMA/PTSD study. He began publishing in medical journals on the subject of psychedelics as a trainee and since then has spoken nationally and internationally to doctors in a campaign to see these fascinating substances return to the mainstream pharmacopeia where their lives began. In 2008 he became a Research Associate under Prof. David Nutt at Bristol University, where he consulted for the ACMD on MDMA before working on the UK's only human hallu-cinogen study in modern times – being the first person to be legally admin-istered a classical psychedelic drug in this country for 33 years.

Sjöstedt-H, Peter: Peter is an Anglo-Scandinavian philosopher who spe-cialises in the thought of Schopenhauer, Nietzsche, and Bergson, within the field of Philosophy of Mind. Peter has a Bachelor's degree in Philoso-phy and a Master's degree in Continental Philosophy from the University of Warwick, where he was awarded a first-class distinction for his dis-sertation on Kant and Schelling in relation to 'intellectual intuition'. Peter subsequently became a philosophy lecturer in South Kensington, London for six years before returning to the tranquillity of westernmost Cornwall with his partner and young son. He is now an independent philosopher, giving talks around Europe while writing essays, articles and a forthcom-ing book. He can be contacted via facebook.com/ontologistics or youtube.com/ontologistics – or by email at peter@philosopher.eu

Slater, Toby: Toby Slater is a politics and philosophy graduate with eclec-tic interests in sociology, anthropology, spirituality, creativity; and the role and therapeutic potential of psychedelics. Toby currently works as a guid-ance practitioner for a youth homelessness prevention project in West Sus-sex. His creative work includes a literary-fiction novel; poetry; lyrics; and freelance articles and essays for various organisations including The Beck-ley Foundation. Toby is also a singer-songwriter who writes and performs.

Strassman, Rick: Rick Strassman MD is Clinical Associate Professor of Psychiatry, University of New Mexico, School of Medicine. He is the author of *DMT: The Spirit Molecule* and *DMT and the Soul of Prophecy*. His website is rickstrassman.com

Yellow, About: About Yellow is a twenty-something, Cambridge English lit graduate and gardener who exiled herself from Britain in favour of Berlin. She has written a couple of plays and performs poetry, and also has a rarely updated blog: aboutyellow.blogspot.com. Her addiction is to youth and our generation. Life is currently a farm in Botswana were she is learning to keep bees and grow cacti.

Index